Quick-Fix
Massage

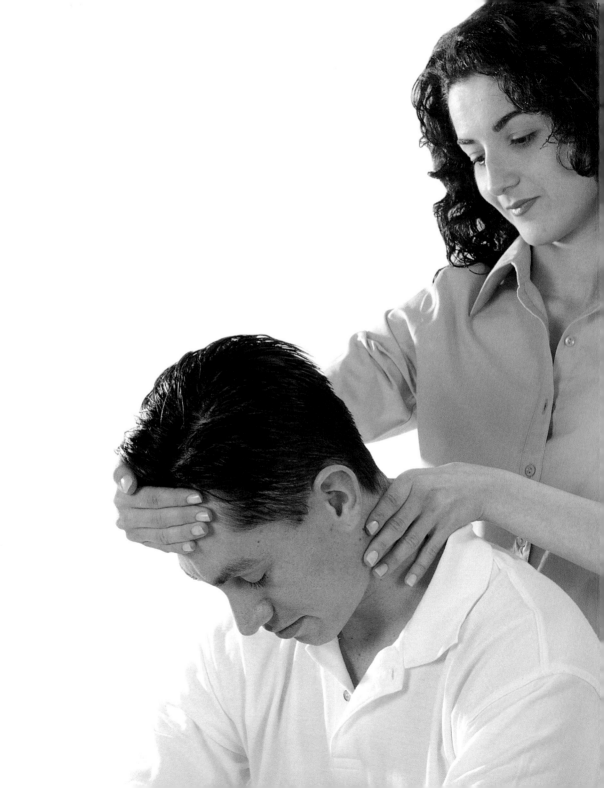

Quick-Fix
Massage

Simple Ways
to Relieve Head,
Neck & Shoulder
Tension

Nitya Lacroix

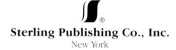

Sterling Publishing Co., Inc.
New York

To my sister, Mary

Please Note

This book is not intended as guidance for the diagnosis or treatment of serious health
problems; please refer to a medical professional if you are in any doubt about any aspect of
your condition. The author, packager and publisher cannot be held responsible for any
injuries which may result from the use of information in this book.

AN EDDISON • SADD EDITION

Edited, designed and produced by Eddison Sadd Editions Limited
St Chad's House, 148 King's Cross Road
London WC1X 9DH

Text copyright © Nitya Lacroix 2002
Photographs copyright © Sue Atkinson 2002
This edition copyright © Eddison Sadd Editions 2002

Library of Congress
Cataloging-in-Publication Available

1   3   5   7   9   10   8   6   4   2

Published in 2002 by Sterling Publishing Company, Inc.
387 Park Avenue South, New York, N.Y. 10016

Distributed in Canada by Sterling Publishing
c/o Canadian Manda Group
One Atlantic Avenue, Suite 106
Toronto, Ontario, Canada, M6K 3E7

Phototypeset in Bell Gothic BT, Franklin Gothic BT and
P22 Vincent using QuarkXPress on Apple Macintosh
Origination by Pixel Graphics, Singapore
Printed and bound by Star Standard Industries (PTE Ltd), Singapore

Sterling ISBN 0-8069-8943-2

Contents

Introduction

Most people experience back, shoulder or neck discomfort at some point in their lives. Although often manifested as little more than a niggling ache and some stiffness in the joints and muscles, the pain may sometimes cause real problems and a reduction or loss of mobility in these areas. The back and spine are the key structures of support in the human body, so back pain, whether acute or chronic, minor or severe, can leave you feeling emotionally and physically drained.

We all want to function at our best for work, but every year millions of working days are lost through sick-leave due to back pain. This results in a significant amount of lost production and income annually. However, can be the demands of work that cause these afflictions in the first place. Pressure of work, poor posture while sitting at a desk, factory line or supermarket check out repetitive movements and other strains, both mental and physical, cause muscles to tighten, and instigate wear and tear on the body's ligaments, tendons and joints.

The quick-fix techniques in this book focus on the upper back, shoulders and neck – a region that is prone to accumulating tension through work-related stress. Suggestions are given as to how to implement a morning-to-night care routine that encourages you to take note of how and where tension is gathering during the day. It also provides a variety of ways to dispel this tension quickly and without fuss, both at home and at work, through its easy yet comprehensive programme of exercise, massage and postural-awareness techniques.

The book features instruction on working on yourself and on work colleagues. This can be done using the hands-on methods described, or using a massage tool, as shown in the information panels throughout the book.

A morning-to-night programme

The six chapters of this book show you how to create a programme of self-care, from the moment you rise to the minute you go to bed, so that your neck and shoulders remain free of tension throughout the day.

The basic manual strokes of Swedish massage are explained in Chapter One to help you construct a quick stress-reducing massage for work colleagues, or a soothing massage to be enjoyed at leisure in the comfort of your home. Follow the early-morning routine of self-massage and gentle exercise suggested in Chapter

Two to start each day feeling invigorated and refreshed. Chapter Three offers tips on maintaining good posture and describes an exercise and self-massage programme for your work breaks, while Chapter Four encourages you to exchange 'quick-fix' massages with your colleagues, by describing the appropriate use of a massage tool as well as manual massage techniques in an office environment. The last two chapters provide ideas for relaxation at home. Chapter Five explains passive movement techniques, which are designed to relieve both psychological and physical tension. Finally, Chapter Six reveals the strokes of a wonderfully soothing neck, head and face massage to help you unwind from the stresses of the day so you can enjoy a relaxed evening and a calm sleep.

The anatomy of the upper body

Some basic knowledge of the anatomy of the upper back will help you to understand why it is so important to maintain a good posture and to ensure your neck and shoulders remain relaxed and flexible throughout the day. By visualizing the complex and interrelated structures of this region, you will learn how harmful postural habits cause muscular tension and stress on the bones, and increase wear and tear on the joints, tendons and ligaments.

Muscles and joints

The main groups of muscles on which this book focuses are largely involved with the movement of the head, neck, shoulders and arms. Like all muscles, they are attached to areas of bone by tendons. A tendon is a white fibrous cord of flexible tissue which connects muscle to bone, or muscle to muscle. Movement takes place when a muscle contracts and puts pressure on the tendon which, in turn, draws one attached bone towards the other. The muscles in the neck and upper back are responsible for the movements of the head, whether it is turning from side to side, elevating, or flexing and extending. The head-moving muscles are attached at one end to the side or base of the skull and, at the other, to the spine, shoulder blade or collarbone. In order to support the upright position of the head, these muscles must always retain a degree of tension. It is important, however, that this tension is not unduly exaggerated, as can occur through stress or bad posture.

Most of the muscles in the shoulder girdle region originate from and stabilize the shoulder blades, and are responsible for the considerable, free and varied movements of the shoulder blades, shoulder joints and arms. Nine muscles traverse the shoulder joint. Four of them are deep muscles with tendons that encapsulate the

Upper-body muscles

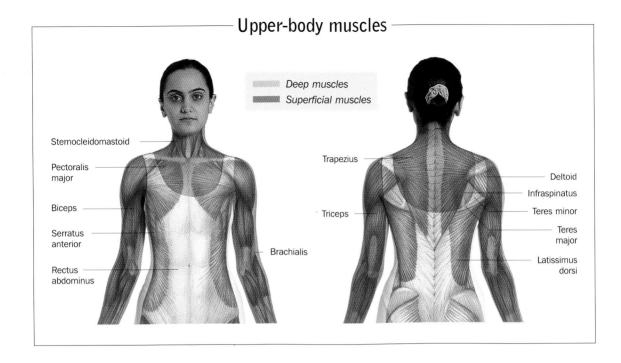

Deep muscles
Superficial muscles

Sternocleidomastoid

Pectoralis major

Biceps

Serratus anterior

Rectus abdominus

Brachialis

Trapezius

Triceps

Deltoid

Infraspinatus

Teres minor

Teres major

Latissimus dorsi

joint; this group, known as the 'rotator cuff', is a common site of injury or pain from strain, wear and tear. Inflammation can also occur in the tendons of these deep muscles.

Joints are the connection points between bones. Without them, it would be impossible for the bones of the body to move. Most joints have considerable mobility (for example, the shoulder joint), some have a small degree of movement (for example, the spinal vertebrae), while others are fused or fixed (the skull). Joints are bound to the bone by ligaments which are composed

of strong, elastic, fibrous tissue. The role of ligaments is to stabilize the joint and all its movements. Non-specific back and neck pain is often due to ligament strain. This, in turn, is exacerbated by tense muscles that pull on the bones and restrict the blood flow which, otherwise, keeps tissues oxygenated and healthy.

The spine

The neck is part of the spine, the bones, or vertebrae, of which protect the central nervous system within the spinal cord. They also provide the

Shoulder and spine

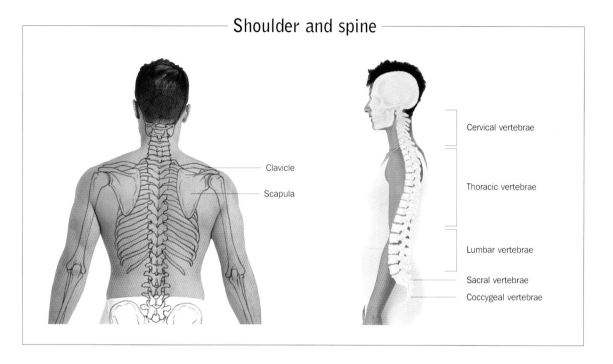

Clavicle

Scapula

Cervical vertebrae

Thoracic vertebrae

Lumbar vertebrae

Sacral vertebrae

Coccygeal vertebrae

main support structure of the body. Thirty-three bones make up the spinal column. Of these, twenty-four are separate; they form the major part of the spine, from the top of the neck to the lower back. Then there are five fused vertebrae, which form the 'sacrum' (the flat, triangular bone at the base of the back), and four fused vertebrae, the coccyx, which make up the tailbone. Of the moveable bones, the neck consists of seven cervical vertebrae, the middle region of the back has twelve thoracic vertebrae, and there are five lumbar, or lower-back, bones.

The spine has four natural curves. The curves in the neck and lower back form in early infancy from the actions of lifting the head and standing. The thoracic curve of the middle back and the sacral curve of the tailbone are retained from the curled foetal position in the womb. These curves safeguard the health of the spine, as they absorb shock from everyday movements, such as walking and running, and from accidents such as falls. In addition, they increase the strength and flexibility of the spine and help the body to remain in an upright and balanced position. Good posture helps to maintain the spine's natural curvature. When seated for long periods, avoid slumping or dropping your head forward as this will reduce natural curvature, straining the spine and adjoining muscles, tendons and ligaments.

The twenty-four moveable bones of the spine, which are smaller in the neck and increase in size in the lumbar region, are connected to each other by inter-vertebral discs. These consist of an outer ring of fibrous tissue and an inner core of a jelly-like substance and they act like joints, permitting flexibility in the spine and enabling it to accomplish its backwards, forwards and side-ways movements. They also serve to protect the vertebrae from shock and injury. The discs and vertebrae are bound together by strong liga-ments and supported by thread-like muscles.

The first two bones of the cervical vertebrae vary in shape and structure from the rest of the spinal column. The one immediately below the skull is called the atlas, and is a ring shape. It has joints that attach to the base of the skull and permit the nodding, or 'yes', gesture of the head. The second cervical vertebra, called the axis, has an upward tooth-like protrusion that fits into the atlas to form a pivot joint, which allows the head to make a side-to-side rotation, or the 'no' gesture. The bones of the neck support the weight of the head (approximately 6.3kg/14lb), and are capable of the greatest degree of flexi-bility in the whole spine. If the neck stiffens, then the natural movements of the head can become severely restricted.

The flexibility of the two shoulder girdle is also important. Each consists of the collarbone (clavicle), which attaches to the breastbone (sternum), the shoulder blade (scapula), which is secured to the spine by muscles, and the long bone of the upper arm (humerus). The collarbone and shoulder blade form the bony part of the shoulder. The top bone of the arm fits into a cavity on the shoulder blade just below the junction with the collarbone, forming the shoulder joint.

How injury occurs

The complexity of the network of muscles, tendons, bones, joints and ligaments of the neck, shoulders and spine is the reason why tension in one area may result in injury in another. Tight or overworked muscles between the shoulder blades may cause pain and restrict movement in the shoulder joints and arms. Pressure on nerves leaving the upper spine can result in referred pain, numbness or tingling in the arm and fingers. A stiff neck or tight face muscles may lead to a tension headache and eye-strain.

The main question is why does undue tension or injury occur in the neck and upper back in the first place? The answer may be as simple as inadequate bedding, such as a mattress or pillow which are failing to give proper support and alignment to the spine or comfort to your body while you sleep (see Chapter Two). Sitting in a draught, or damp, cold weather, may cause the neck muscles to stiffen. Undertaking sudden strenuous activity, such as certain sports, gardening and decorating, may overwork and injure tendons and ligaments, especially if you are not supple and fit beforehand. One of the most likely culprits of upper-back pain is poor posture, particularly if you are overworked and have to sit for long hours leaning over a desk, or your work involves repetitive movements (see Chapter Three).

Emotional stress is also a trigger for muscular tension in the shoulders, neck and upper back. If you feel burdened, under pressure, angry or sad, a common reaction is to hunch up or curl in your shoulders and tighten your face and back muscles as a form of protection or a way to suppress uncomfortable feelings. It is vitally important to relax psychologically as well as physically. No matter how busy you are, or how upset you are, take time to do things that you enjoy, such as having a massage, walking, swimming, dancing or just relaxing with friends. Try to understand the causes of your anxieties and find constructive ways to change things for the better.

Avoiding problems

Good posture is vital to the health of your spine and muscle condition. Always try to carry the concept of length and width in your body, allowing your spine to extend upwards naturally and gracefully, so that your head is elevated and balanced over the spine, and there is a feeling of width and space in your upper back, chest and shoulders. Visualize your arms as lengthening down from your shoulders. Avoid slumping in your spine, hunching or bracing your shoulders, straining forward, dropping your head, or jutting out your jaw. Consciously stop, check and relax your posture throughout the day.

Whether you are in the motion of walking, or you are standing or sitting, the image of length and width in your upper body should always be with you.

Getting help

Most neck and shoulder problems are uncomfortable and debilitating but are usually not serious and are likely to disappear of their own accord within days or weeks. Before starting any self-help programme, however, it is advisable to check with your doctor. If you follow the gentle exercise and massage programmes in this book, you should be able to reduce the likelihood of accumulating serious tension in the tissues and increase flexibility in these areas.

If you suffer from neck and shoulder pain, there are several ways to relieve it at home. Tight and strained muscles respond well to heat treatment. Soak the afflicted area as you relax in a warm bath or apply a heated compress in the form of a wrapped hot water bottle or a special heating pad, taking care to protect your skin. Heat works by increasing the blood flow to the sore area, which aids recovery and repair of strained ligaments and muscles. An ice pack can be used to treat tension headaches, or applied to inflamed and sprained areas to reduce swelling and bruising and limit further tissue damage. Use a specially designed ice pack or simply wrap ice-cubes or a pack of frozen peas in a cloth.

Some neck and shoulder pain is indicative of more serious injury, a chronic disorder, or a degenerative condition in the spine. As we get older, there is an inevitable process of wear and tear on the joints and vertebrae. The inter-vertebral discs sometimes shrink and the bones thicken. Bony protrusions can grow out of the discs and adversely affect the joints. If the pain persists and is severe or is causing numbness or nerve sensation, you should seek the advice of your doctor. You may be referred to a physiotherapist who can show you appropriate exercises or who may apply heat treatment to the afflicted tissues, possibly using infrared wave lamps, ultrasound or laser therapy. Your doctor may also prescribe a short course of anti-inflammatory medication or refer you on to an orthopaedic hospital consultant for further investigation.

Complementary therapies can also be of great benefit. Massage, except in the case of acute and severe pain or swelling, is very helpful in soothing tension from the body and relaxing the mind. An aromatherapy massage may involve the use of essential oils renowned for their warming, relaxing and healing properties. Acupuncture has an excellent reputation in the treatment of ligament and tendon injuries, or you may wish to consult a qualified and registered osteopath or chiropractitioner who is specifically trained in the prevention and treatment of spinal and muscular disorders. Most of

Massage tools

You may find it helpful to buy a massage tool for some of these routines, particularly for massaging in places where there is no privacy or on someone you don't know very well. These come in a variety of shapes and sizes as shown below, and are specially designed to manipulate tight spots on the body to release tension and boost blood flow. A shape such as that shown bottom left, which is used throughout this book, is particularly versatile as its pegs can be individually manipulated to apply different amounts of pressure to different parts of the body.

By pressing or rolling the tool, you can quickly invigorate your own body and relieve stiffness and discomfort. A self-applied massage, rolled or pressed against muscles in the head, neck, shoulders and arms, brings release. In addition, a massage tool works wonders when applied to hands, legs and feet.

all, develop a healthy body consciousness, so that you can become quickly aware of pain and tension in your body, especially in those vital areas of the neck, shoulders and spine. Do not take your body for granted or treat it like a machine, and do not ignore pain and discomfort. Tension, whether it is physical or emotional, can be quickly dispelled if you pay attention to its causes and take measures to relax yourself or the situation. Respect your body and nurture it no matter how pressing external demands may be. Take adequate exercise and rest, maintain a healthy diet, and inform yourself of ways to seek relief and comfort from stress and pain.

Remember, however, that your most important ally in maintaining a pain-free and relaxed body is yourself. Follow the simple instructions in this book to enjoy being 'head and shoulders' above tension, no matter how busy you are at work.

Basic massage strokes

An effective massage is one that results in both physical and mental relaxation, while also leaving the recipient feeling refreshed and invigorated. To achieve this, a massage should involve a variety of strokes that follow a certain sequence. The initial strokes should soothe and relax a body area by warming and easing the tissues. Once the muscles start to soften under the rhythmic and flowing motion of hands on the skin, it becomes possible to apply stronger strokes to manipulate muscles, boost the blood circulation or grind into tight spots for a deeper release of tension. Finally, the massage should be completed with a return to softer strokes or a gentle hold to encourage a calm sense of body and mind equilibrium. The basic strokes described in this chapter are taken from the techniques of Swedish massage, which form the basis of many massage styles. You are shown how to apply them to the upper back area, including the neck and shoulders, which is the focus of this book. These strokes, however, can be applied to all areas of the body when and where it is appropriate to do so, and can be adapted to form a self-massage.

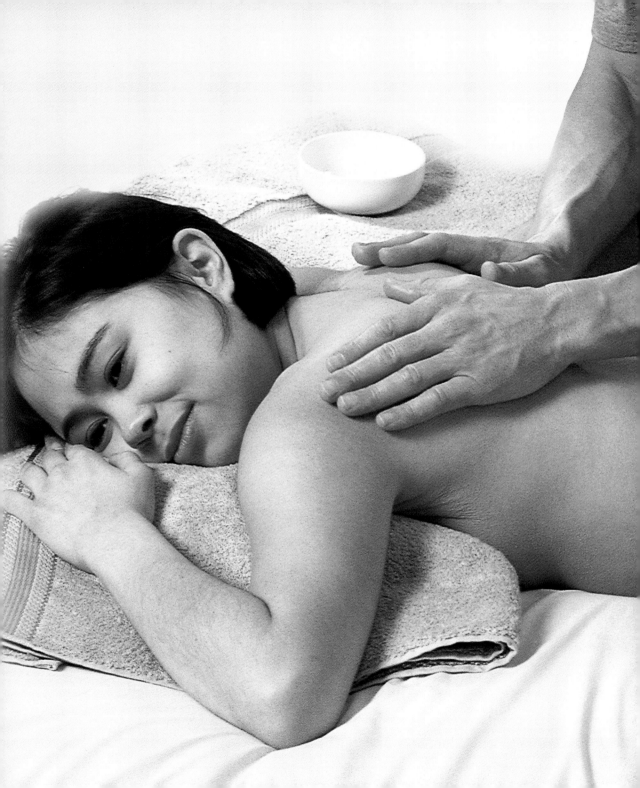

Effleurage strokes

Effleurage strokes are smooth and flowing and are applied from the flat surface of the palms and fingers of the hands. These strokes have a steady, hypnotic rhythm, which allows both the giver and receiver time to relax. When performing effleurage strokes, your hands should be firm but soft, moulding to the body shape and not imposing on it. These movements warm and stretch the superficial tissues of the body, easing tension from underlying muscles and increasing blood flow to the area. Their continuous rounded motions are pleasant, soporific and calming to the nervous system and the mind, creating a holistic mental and physical relaxation, while preparing the muscles for more vigorous techniques. The fan stroke, which is described below, is an effleurage movement that can be adapted to be used on the torso and limbs. Here, it encompasses and releases tension from the upper back. Each sequence of effleurage strokes can be repeated three times before performing the next motion.

The fan stroke

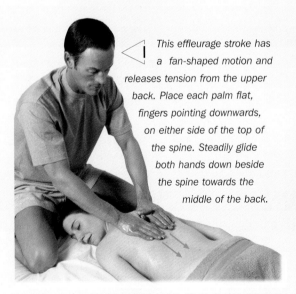

1 This effleurage stroke has a fan-shaped motion and releases tension from the upper back. Place each palm flat, fingers pointing downwards, on either side of the top of the spine. Steadily glide both hands down beside the spine towards the middle of the back.

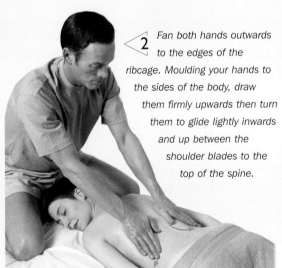

2 Fan both hands outwards to the edges of the ribcage. Moulding your hands to the sides of the body, draw them firmly upwards then turn them to glide lightly inwards and up between the shoulder blades to the top of the spine.

Basic massage tips

When doing a massage, ensure that your environment is warm, private, calming and comfortable. If the person receiving the massage is lying down, it should be on a supportive surface such as a mattress or futon. Use towels to cover parts of the body not being massaged to prevent the body temperature from dropping. When giving a massage, take care of your posture, keeping your spine and neck lengthened and your shoulders widened. If you are kneeling on the mattress, try placing one foot on the surface to give

yourself support and greater scope of movement. Lubricating the area you are about to work on will ensure an easy flow of motion with your hands. This can be done using an unrefined cold-pressed vegetable oil, such as grapeseed or sunflower, enriched by adding a few drops of almond or avocado oil, or a ready-made shop-bought massage oil. Use a plastic oil container that will emit a few drops at a time. Rub the oil into the palms of your hands to warm it before massaging it on your partner's body.

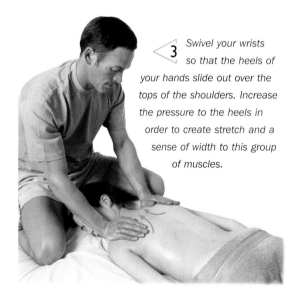

3 Swivel your wrists so that the heels of your hands slide out over the tops of the shoulders. Increase the pressure to the heels in order to create stretch and a sense of width to this group of muscles.

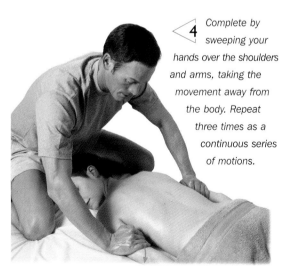

4 Complete by sweeping your hands over the shoulders and arms, taking the movement away from the body. Repeat three times as a continuous series of motions.

Circle strokes

Circle strokes are effleurage motions that follow on perfectly from the initial fan strokes. They are rounded, flowing movements that warm the skin and lightly stretch the underlying tissue. In addition, they are wonderfully relaxing. Apply them to the broader surface areas of the body. Here they are shown on the upper back, but they can be used equally well on the lower back, buttocks, thighs and stomach. The circular stroke is applied as a continuous spiralling motion to cover the area you are massaging. Your hands need to be co-ordinated as the stroke requires the left hand to make a continuous clockwise motion on the body, while the right hand lifts up to let the left hand pass beneath it before returning to complete a half-circle movement. Both hands should work closely together to form a succinct circular shape while in motion. The speed and pressure of the circle stroke can be varied. The lighter and slower the stroke, the more relaxing it is. Firmer pressure and faster movement is more invigorating. Do the circle strokes on the side of the body furthest from you, keeping your arms outstretched but with elbows flexed and wrists relaxed.

Place your hands side by side, but slightly apart, on the side of the body at the base of the ribcage. Start to circle both hands in a clockwise motion.

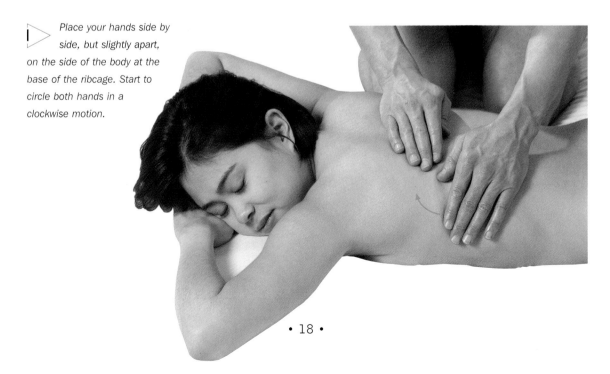

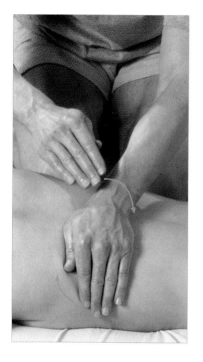

2 Lift the right hand off the body and pass it over the wrist of the left hand as it slides underneath and continues to complete the circular movement.

3 Drop the right hand back down on to the body so that it completes a semi-circular motion, before lifting up again and passing over the continuously moving left hand. Slowly spiral the circle strokes up along the ribcage, sliding your hands on to the shoulder blade to circulate several times over it before continuing the motion down alongside the spine. Do this sequence three times, then repeat on the other side of the body.

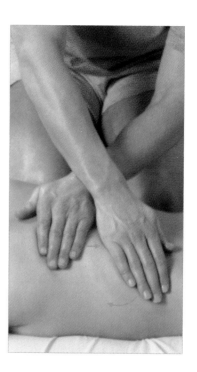

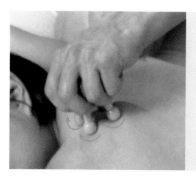

Massage-tool circles

A massage tool can also be used to make soothing circular motions over the back and shoulder blades. Rotate the pegs in continuous and spiralling circles up along the ribcage, several times over the surface of the shoulder blade, and down beside the spine. Repeat the sequence several times before doing the same on the other side of the body.

Kneading strokes

Kneading is one of the most active and effective strokes of massage. Its scooping, squeezing and rolling motion manipulates muscles, breaks down tension and increases circulation to the tissues, while eliminating the waste products that are deposited in them. Kneading strokes bring relief and invigoration to tight spots, such as the shoulders, and to fleshy areas such as the arms. Knead in a continuous rolling, rather than plucking, fashion.

Perform kneading by lifting a portion of flesh away from the body and squeezing it between the fingers and the heel and thumb of one hand as you pass it towards your other hand. Repeat the motion back and forth between the two hands so that the area softens up under the continuously flowing movement. While kneading, keep your elbows flexed and wrists loose, and work on the side of the body opposite to you. Then repeat the strokes on the other side.

Kneading the shoulder

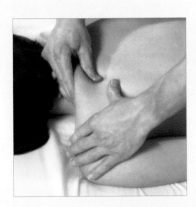 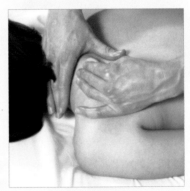 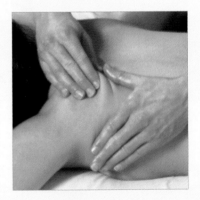

△1△ Adapt the stroke to fit the narrow area of the shoulder by lifting and squeezing the flesh between the fingers and thumb of one hand before rolling it towards the other hand.

△2△ Receive the roll of flesh with the second hand. Lift, wring and then push it back towards the passive hand. Perform this rolling motion back and forth to soften the muscles that surround the base of the neck.

△△ KNEADING THE UPPER BODY Knead up the side of the ribcage, alongside and over the shoulder blade, and on to the top of the arm.

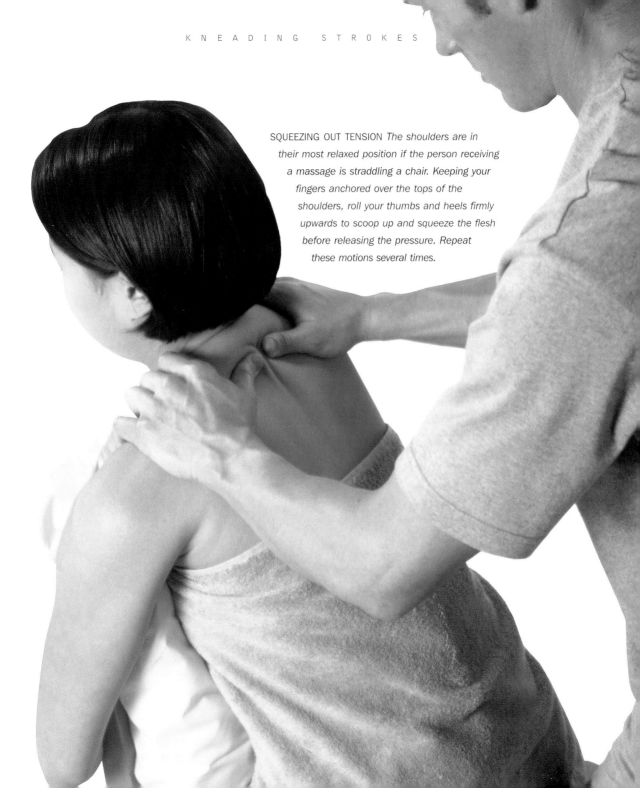

SQUEEZING OUT TENSION *The shoulders are in their most relaxed position if the person receiving a massage is straddling a chair. Keeping your fingers anchored over the tops of the shoulders, roll your thumbs and heels firmly upwards to scoop up and squeeze the flesh before releasing the pressure. Repeat these motions several times.*

Petrissage strokes

Petrissage is a grinding stroke that releases a deeper layer of tension in the body. It is particularly effective when used in small or tight areas that surround bone, making it an ideal stroke to apply to the base of the neck, between the shoulder blades and alongside the spine. Once an area of the body has been warmed and relaxed through effleurage and kneading strokes, petrissage can be applied by using pressure from your fingers or thumbs or the heels of the hands. With petrisssage strokes the pressure should always be applied at a slow and steady pace so as not to jar the muscle. Sink your fingers or thumbs gradually into the tissue to a depth that is comfortable to the massage recipient. Petrissage may take the

Petrissage along the spine

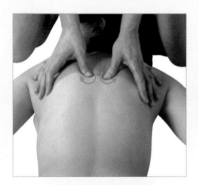

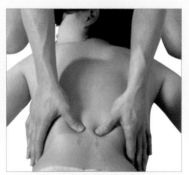

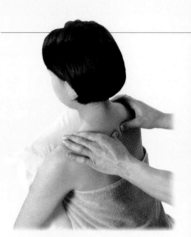

△ CIRCULAR PETRISSAGE *Use circular petrissage strokes down the long muscles that support the spine. Resting both hands lightly on the back, sink both thumbs into the area at each side of the top of the spine. Make small spiralling rotations with both thumbs downward to the mid-back. Repeat three times.*

△ SLIDING PETRISSAGE *Press your thumbs gently into the muscles on each side of the top of the spine. Lean your weight into your thumbs to apply a slow, firm, sliding motion either side of the spine towards the mid-back. Repeat the sequence three times and then soothe the back with fan strokes.*

△ PETRISSAGING TIGHT AREAS *Petrissage is perfect for alleviating tension from between the shoulder blades. If your partner is in the sitting position, hook your fingers over the top of the shoulders for anchorage. Rotate your thumbs in the areas between the shoulder blades.*

form of small rotations or of a sliding motion, and the pressure of the stroke should always be released slowly. Always follow up these deeper petrissage strokes with effleurage motions to soothe the area.

When applying circular petrissage rotations from the thumbs, increase the pressure on the inward and downward portion of the circular motion, and decrease the pressure as your thumbs glide out and around. This variation of pressure creates a smoother effect than the circular motion. If you are repeating a series of petrissage strokes, always make sure you return your hands to their original position in a smooth and flowing fashion. For example, if you have completed the circular or sliding petrissage strokes down each side of the spine to the mid-back as shown below, left, glide your palms smoothly up the back of the spine before repeating the sequence.

Petrissage with a massage tool

By applying any degree of pressure using a massage tool, you will automatically perform a petrissage stroke due to the depression of the pegs into the body tissue. Greater depth can be achieved by leaning the weight into just one or two pegs and making small rotations. This works well on the area at the base of the neck and across the tops of the shoulders.

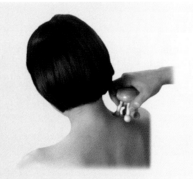

$\triangle$ **1** *The area where the base of the neck joins the shoulder is frequently a sore or tense point. Tip the massager and use the weight of one peg to rotate over this spot several times, gradually increasing the pressure as the tissue softens.*

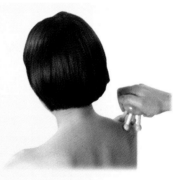

$\triangle$ **2** *Using just two pegs of the massager, circulate the tool thoroughly over the top of the shoulder from the neck to the shoulder joint. Decrease the pressure over the bone. Repeat these two strokes on the other side of the body.*

Percussion strokes

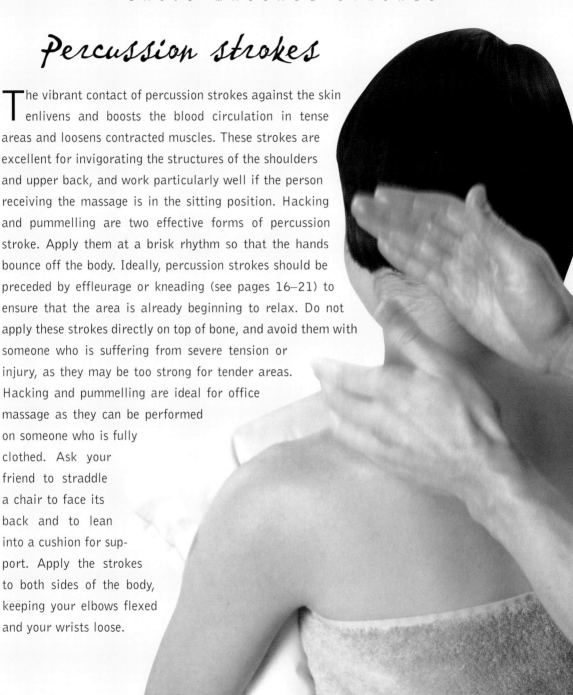

The vibrant contact of percussion strokes against the skin enlivens and boosts the blood circulation in tense areas and loosens contracted muscles. These strokes are excellent for invigorating the structures of the shoulders and upper back, and work particularly well if the person receiving the massage is in the sitting position. Hacking and pummelling are two effective forms of percussion stroke. Apply them at a brisk rhythm so that the hands bounce off the body. Ideally, percussion strokes should be preceded by effleurage or kneading (see pages 16–21) to ensure that the area is already beginning to relax. Do not apply these strokes directly on top of bone, and avoid them with someone who is suffering from severe tension or injury, as they may be too strong for tender areas. Hacking and pummelling are ideal for office massage as they can be performed on someone who is fully clothed. Ask your friend to straddle a chair to face its back and to lean into a cushion for support. Apply the strokes to both sides of the body, keeping your elbows flexed and your wrists loose.

Hacking

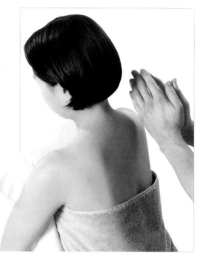

◁ HACKING THE SHOULDERS *Let your palms face each other a* short distance apart. Your fingers should be straight and relaxed. Bounce the sides of your hands, one after the other, across the top of the shoulders.

▷ DOUBLE-HANDED HACKING *Put your hands lightly together.* Rhythmically drum the sides of the hands simultaneously to invigorate the top of the shoulders. This can also be done briskly over the scalp using a lighter pressure.

Pummelling

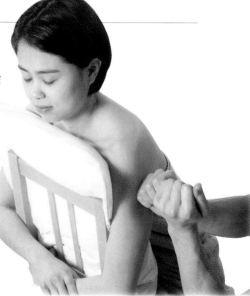

◁ PUMMELLING THE SHOULDERS *Pummelling is done by making* loose fists of your hands and drumming them, one after the other, over muscular areas of the body such as the shoulders.

▷ PUMMELLING THE ARMS *Pummel over the tops of* the arms to boost circulation. This can also ease the tension which surrounds the shoulder joints and bring greater flexibility to the movement of the arms.

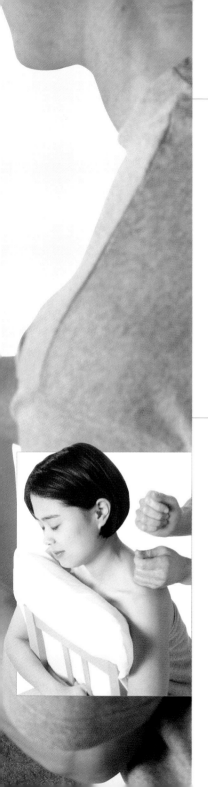

Using a massager with a partner

A massager, such as that described in the Introduction (page 13), can be used in place of traditional hands-on strokes when massaging a partner or friend. While a mechanical aid cannot replicate the healing quality of touch that comes from the direct physical contact of hands on the body, it can still provide the right amount of pressure, friction and stimulation to relax muscles and alleviate tension. Some people may even be more comfortable receiving a mechanical massage rather than a manual one.

You can also use a massager if you are not yet confident with applying the more complicated techniques of manual strokes, or if you do not have the physical energy to give a full-body tactile massage. The pleasant sensation of the motion of the massager's pegs against the body will be enhanced if a small amount of lotion is first applied to the skin. Always depress the pegs into the tissue at a slow and steady pace, so as not to jar the muscle. Repeat the movements described here on both sides of the body.

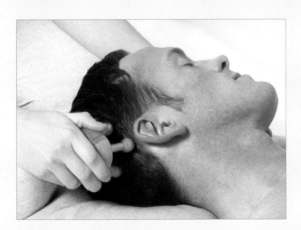

△ HEAD MASSAGE *Tilt the head, first into the palm of one hand, and then the other, in order to apply the massager to all sides of its circumference. Apply invigorating small circles to one area at a time, before sliding the pegs on to the adjoining surface of scalp.*

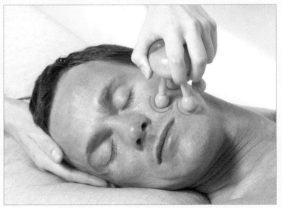

△ FACE MASSAGE *Leaning the pressure lightly into the massager's front pegs, ease tension from the forehead, cheeks and jaw with small outward-flowing rotary motions. Heed the natural contours of the face, working sensitively around areas of bone.*

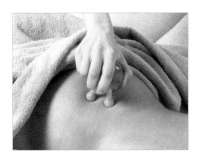

△ FLESHY AREAS *The massager is at its most effective when applied to the more fleshy parts of the body, such as the buttocks and thighs. Initially, flowing circular motions should be made to relax the muscles. Follow these up with small, invigorating rotations which enliven the tissue.*

▷ THE TORSO *Circulate the massager on the side opposite to you and make a continuous spiralling motion. Start from the lower back, moving up beside the spine, over the shoulder blade and down the side of the ribcage. Repeat several times.*

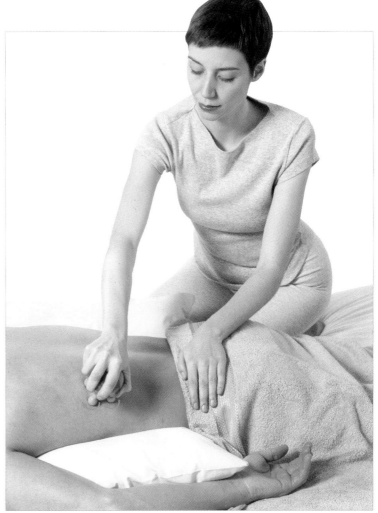

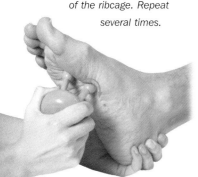

◁ SOLES OF FEET *Ensuring that your partner's leg is comfortable, and the knee supported and flexed, work the massager over the sole of the foot to alleviate tension. Tip the tool to focus the* weight onto two pegs and indent steadily into one area at a time, turning the pegs in a clockwise semi-circular motion. Release the pressure before moving to the next spot.

Basic strokes for self-massage

All of the basic techniques described in this chapter can be combined and adapted to create a satisfying self-massage. Through these strokes you can learn how to dispel tension wherever it accumulates in your body. Self-massage will increase your awareness of your own body and encourage you to take good care of your well-being on a regular basis. Repeat the strokes described here on both sides of the body.

Use it first thing in the morning, to stimulate nerve endings and enliven your whole system for the day ahead. Apply the strokes in the evening to relax tired, tense areas of your body and to massage away stress.

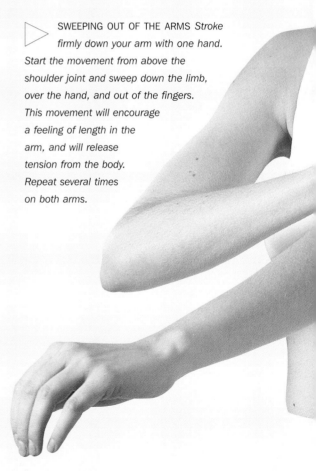

▷ SWEEPING OUT OF THE ARMS *Stroke firmly down your arm with one hand. Start the movement from above the shoulder joint and sweep down the limb, over the hand, and out of the fingers. This movement will encourage a feeling of length in the arm, and will release tension from the body. Repeat several times on both arms.*

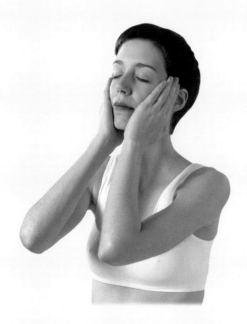

◁ SOOTHING STROKES *Circulate the smooth surface of your palms and fingers several times over your forehead, cheeks and jaw to relax your face. Follow up these effleurage strokes by sweeping your fingertips several times over your temples.*

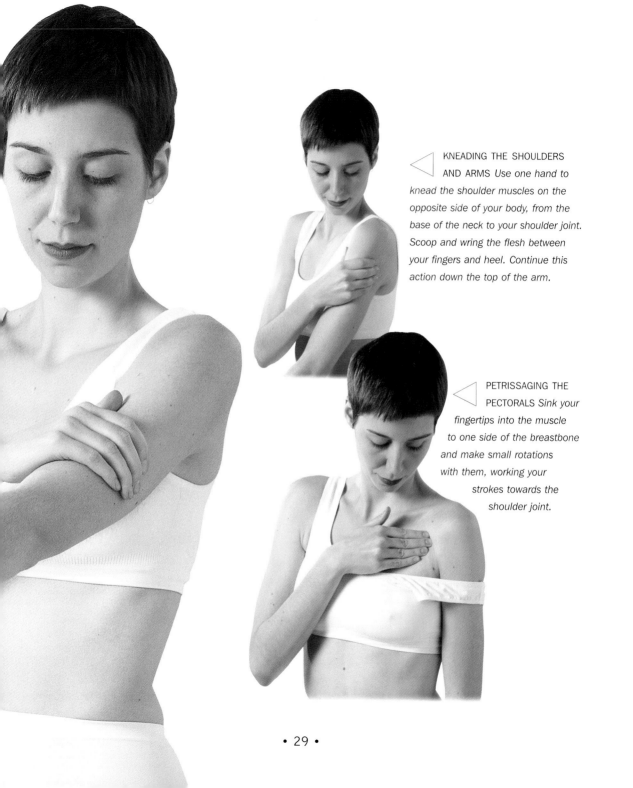

KNEADING THE SHOULDERS AND ARMS *Use one hand to knead the shoulder muscles on the opposite side of your body, from the base of the neck to your shoulder joint. Scoop and wring the flesh between your fingers and heel. Continue this action down the top of the arm.*

PETRISSAGING THE PECTORALS *Sink your fingertips into the muscle to one side of the breastbone and make small rotations with them, working your strokes towards the shoulder joint.*

• 29 •

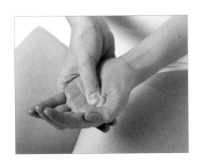

△ PETRISSAGING THE HANDS
*Short, sliding petrissage
strokes, made with the thumb of one
hand all over the palm of the other,
are a good method of stretching and
relaxing your hands. Support the back
of the receptive hand in the palm of
the working hand.*

▷ PUMMELLING THE SHOULDERS
*Make a loose fist with one
hand and use it to thoroughly
pummel the back of the neck,
shoulder and upper arm on the
opposite side of the body. Lift and
support the active arm by holding
its flexed elbow in the palm of the
other hand.*

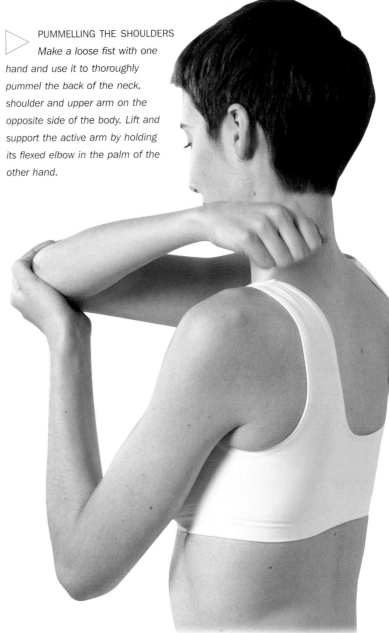

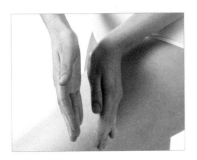

△ HACKING THE THIGHS *Hacking
is an excellent self-massage
stroke to use on the fleshy area of the
thigh. Raise your knee by placing a
foot on a stool or chair, and rapidly
drum the sides of your hands, one
after the other, over the surface of
the upper leg.*

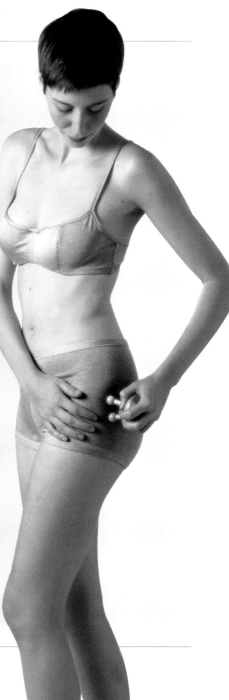

Self-help with a massager

Use a massager at home to stimulate and soothe weary muscles all over your body. Experiment with pressure, speed and size of rotations to find the way you like best to apply to different areas. Tip the tool to work one or two of its pegs into a smaller area or to increase depth. Rubbing a little lotion into your skin beforehand will ensure that it circulates smoothly.

△ SCALP *Apply spiralling circular motions all over your head. Then, to increase stimulation, rotate the pegs in smaller, faster circles.*

▷ HIPS AND BUTTOCKS *By rotating the massager around the hip joint and firmly over the buttock you will invigorate these fleshy areas.*

◁ FEET *Rest your foot on the opposite knee. Focusing pressure into two pegs of the massager, rotate them over the sole to include the base of the toes, the arch and the heel.*

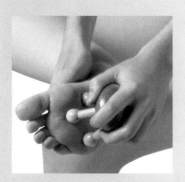

Early-morning exercises

Neck and back pain is so debilitating that it is likely to interfere with how well you function in your job or daily routine. The best way to avoid or alleviate this discomfort is to take preventative action from the start of the day to minimize risk of injury, and reduce and break the insidious cycle of pain and tension. If you are feeling at ease in your body before work, you are less likely to incur a build-up of strain which can result in tight muscles and loss of mobility.

This chapter suggests ways to ensure that the period you spend in bed enhances relaxation and reduces the likelihood of further injury in the upper back area. A short programme of exercise and self-massage, focused on the head, neck and shoulder region, is suggested as a daily early-morning routine to limber up and boost the circulation, and allow greater flexibility and movement in these vital areas. If you start the day with the intention of taking care of your body, this awareness is likely to remain with you as you go through your normal routine.

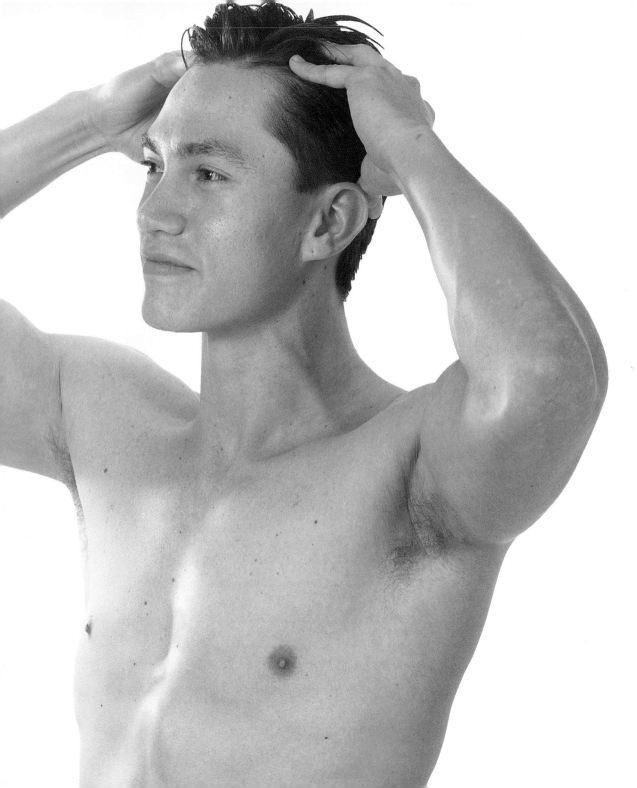

Starting the day relaxed

When you awake, you should feel refreshed and ready to face the demands of the new day. During sleep, body structures, such as the spine, joints, muscles, tendons and ligaments, are able to unwind from stress and release accumulated tensions. Good, sound sleep has a healing and replenishing quality for mind and body and is important for your overall health. Disturbed sleeping patterns or lack of sleep can lead to tension the next day as you will easily become physically weary and find it harder to maintain concentration. You will also have fewer resources to call upon to help you remain alert when under duress. Try to get sufficient sleep to keep your back and spine in good condition, especially during the working week. The quantity of sleep that is needed to function well varies from individual to individual. However, the average person needs seven to eight hours of sleep a night to ensure they have adequate rest.

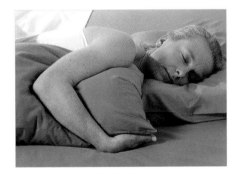

⚠ SLEEPING COMFORTABLY WITH INJURY
Neck and shoulder pain commonly occurs on one side of the body. Sleeping on your good side, rest your head on one pillow and cuddle another pillow so that your injured shoulder relaxes into it and the strain on it is reduced. Flex your knees to relax your spine.

Mattress and pillows

If your muscles feel stiff or painful when you wake, you may need to invest in a good-quality mattress that supports your weight, moulds to your body shape and allows your spine to maintain its natural curves during sleep. The wrong type of mattress, one that is either too soft or too hard, is likely to exacerbate any weaknesses you have in your bones, joints and muscles. Good quality orthopaedic mattresses are designed with back-care in mind, and can be purchased from most bed shops or specialist outlets.

The correct choice of and use of pillows will reduce strain and aid recovery from neck and shoulder injuries. Rest your head on just one pillow during sleep so that your neck remains in line with your spine. Using too many pillows, which raise your head and cause your neck to bend awkwardly, puts additional stress on the spine and shoulder girdle. To reduce this stress on your neck and shoulder region during sleep, you can purchase an orthopaedic pillow. These are specifically designed to cushion your head while keeping your neck aligned to your spine. They are available from specialist back-care shops.

If you are prone to back pain, try sleeping with a pillow behind your knees if you sleep on your back, or between your thighs if you prefer to sleep on your side. Keeping your knees flexed during slumber enables the spine to retain its natural S-curves, relieving strain on the pelvic and neck areas. Avoid sleeping on your stomach as this will cause an uncomfortable twist in your neck and spine.

Take a cue from the way animals rise from sleep, and have a good stretch before getting up. Limber up by gently stretching and flexing your spine, arms and legs. Wiggle your toes and rotate your ankles to get your circulation moving. These movements will stimulate your system and release stiffness before leaving bed.

▽ RISING FROM BED *To arise from bed, roll onto your side to face its edge. Press the hand of your free arm against the surface of the mattress to lever yourself upwards. At the same time, draw your knees towards your body so that you can easily swing your legs off the mattress. Place both feet firmly on the floor and, with relaxed knees, extend your spine, neck and head slowly upwards.*

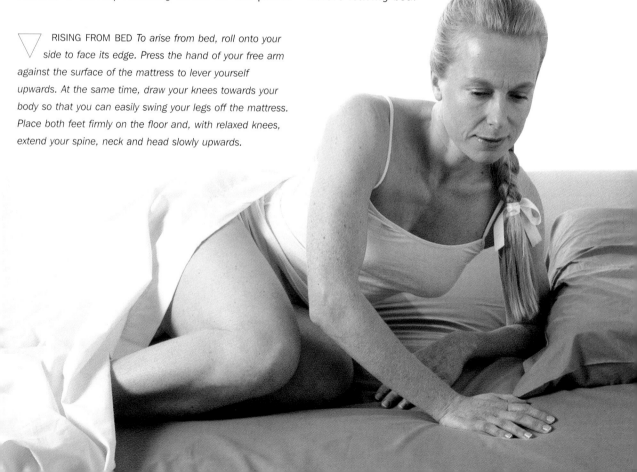

Early-morning exercise routine

Your first stretch of the day should begin while you are still in bed. Limber up with a good all-over stretch, and wiggle your toes and ankles to stimulate your circulation. Once up, implement a routine into your early-morning schedule, allowing yourself time to perform a series of simple stretch exercises and some self-massage before you start your daily tasks. This programme of self-care should take no more than twenty minutes, and will make you feel more relaxed and alert all day.

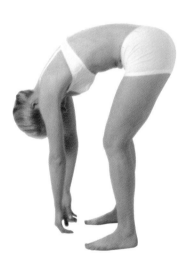

△ STRETCHING UPWARDS
Standing tall, with feet apart, raise your arms upwards so that your fingers stretch up towards the ceiling. This exercise will create extension through your whole body.

△ RELAXING DOWNWARDS *Bend at the knees to lower your hands to the floor. Let your neck and head hang down loosely. Rise by slowly extending your spine to lift your neck and head up last.*

△ SIDE-STRETCH *Stand tall, with your feet shoulder-width apart, and slowly bend your torso to your right, to extend the left ribcage. Return slowly to a standing position and repeat the movement to the left side.*

The stretches and self-massage focus on alleviating tension from your spine, neck and shoulder areas, so that you will be at ease in your movement and posture. Before doing the exercises, try to find the time to take a hot shower to refresh your body and relax your muscles. Aim the shower nozzle at your neck and shoulders in particular, while gently flexing and stretching your upper back area under the stream of warm water.

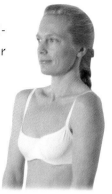

SHOULDER CIRCLES *Circulating your shoulder joints will increase their mobility and ease tension at the base of the neck. Ensuring the motion originates from the joints, rotate your shoulders five times backwards and five times forwards. Repeat three times.*

Holding the stretch

Make sure that you feel as relaxed as possible before starting your routine. If possible do not wear restrictive clothing. Begin by holding the stretches for a count of five, and work up to a count of fifteen as they become more comfortable. Never push, force or bounce any body part against a threshold of tension or pain.

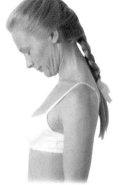

STRETCH TO BACK OF NECK *Drop your chin towards your chest to extend the back of your neck, releasing any contraction in the muscles that support and elevate your head. Then raise your head upwards to a balanced position in line with your spine.*

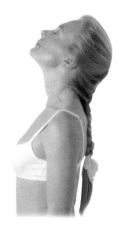

FLEXION TO THE NECK *Following on from the last stretch, slowly drop your head backwards to lengthen the front of your neck, and to cause flexion in the upper vertebrae of the spine. Hold for a moment before returning your head to a balanced position. Repeat this three times, in conjunction with the previous stretch.*

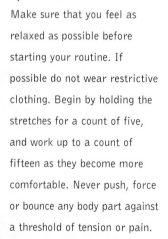

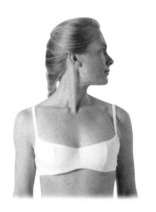

◁ SIDE OF NECK STRETCH
Keeping your shoulders
straight, turn your head
first to the left side and
then to the right side as far
as it feels comfortable to do so and
hold. Repeat this sequence three
times. This eases tension from the
strong muscles each side of the neck.

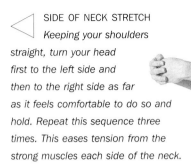

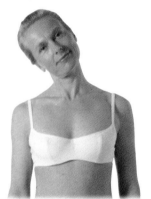

◁ DIAGONAL NECK STRETCH *Tilt*
your head to the right, keeping
your shoulders level so that the left
side of your neck is extended. Hold
the position, then reverse the motion
to the left side. These movements
ease contraction from the muscles at
the base and side of the neck.

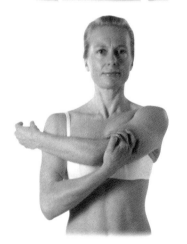

◁ SHOULDER STRETCH *Give the*
back of the shoulder and upper
arm a good stretch by softly clasping a
hand just above the flexed elbow joint
and drawing the arm towards the
opposite shoulder. Then repeat on
the other side.

△ UPPER-BACK STRETCH *Keeping*
your spine lengthened, extend
your arms out in front of you, with
elbows bent and the palm of one hand
resting against the back of the other
hand, and hold this position to stretch
the upper back before relaxing.

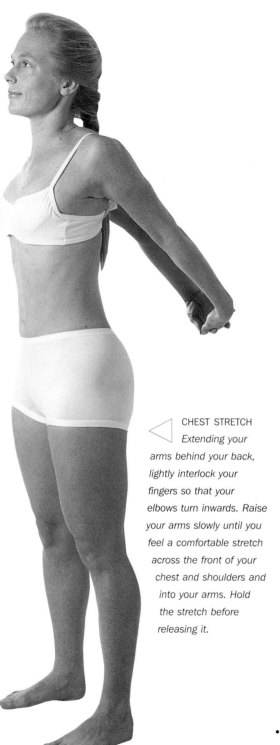

CHEST STRETCH *Extending your arms behind your back, lightly interlock your fingers so that your elbows turn inwards. Raise your arms slowly until you feel a comfortable stretch across the front of your chest and shoulders and into your arms. Hold the stretch before releasing it.*

Face exercises

Stress causes the face to tighten, particularly around the eyes, mouth and jaw. Exercising your facial muscles each morning will loosen these contracted areas, leaving you looking and feeling much more relaxed. This exercise requires you to make 'funny faces', deliberately scrunching up and moving parts of your face to work out the muscles.

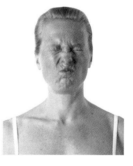

SCRUNCHING THE FACE *Scrunch up your eyes and nose, purse your mouth and wiggle your jaw. Create as much movement in your face muscles as possible for about twenty seconds.*

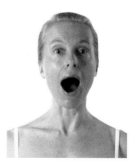

STRETCHING THE FACE *Widen your eyes as far as possible while letting your mouth open and your jaw drop. Hold this position for up to twenty seconds and then relax the muscles.*

Early-morning self-massage

A quick self-massage, focused on the main tension areas in the upper body, will increase physical and mental vitality to give you a good start to the day. The techniques shown here will particularly stimulate the blood circulation while relaxing muscles, leaving you feeling both refreshed and alert. Performing all of these techniques should add no more than ten minutes to your morning schedule.

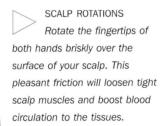

▷ SCALP ROTATIONS
Rotate the fingertips of both hands briskly over the surface of your scalp. This pleasant friction will loosen tight scalp muscles and boost blood circulation to the tissues.

◁ FINGER TAPPING *With a hand on either side of your face, drum your fingertips lightly over your forehead, temples, cheeks and jaw.*

▷ PUMMELLING *Pummel thoroughly down the back of your neck, across the top of the shoulder, down the length of the arm and on to the hand on each side of the body. Support your elbow as you pummel the neck, shoulder and upper arm.*

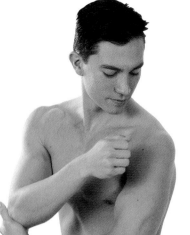

Using a massage tool

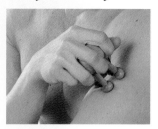

Perform small rotations with the pegs over the muscles beneath the shoulder, and then down the arm and on to the back of the hand. Now work the pegs over the palm and wrist, and up the surface of the inner arm.

▽ SQUEEZING HANDS *Relax your hands by softly squeezing all over one hand with the other and then repeating on the other side. Finally, gently shake your hands.*

◁ BEATING THE CHEST *Briskly pummelling over your chest and pectoral muscles with loose fists will boost the blood flow to the area, relieving tightness to deepen breath and increase the oxygen intake to your lungs.*

CHAPTER THREE

Remaining relaxed at work

Stress is an inevitable aspect of modern working life. Commuting, producing work under pressure and office politics can all create a degree of mental anxiety that leads to physical tension. Long periods of sitting at a desk or making repetitive movements can also put strain on the body, often resulting in pain or injury. In itself, stress can be a motivating factor and is not harmful if you are able to prevent or quickly dispel any tension that it causes in your body. This chapter advises you on how to remain relaxed at work by taking care of your posture and adjusting your working environment so that you protect your body from harm. Tips on exercises, self-massage and breathing techniques, which release both physical and mental tension and can be done discreetly at your desk or during a work break, are given so that you can remain fully active yet relaxed throughout the day.

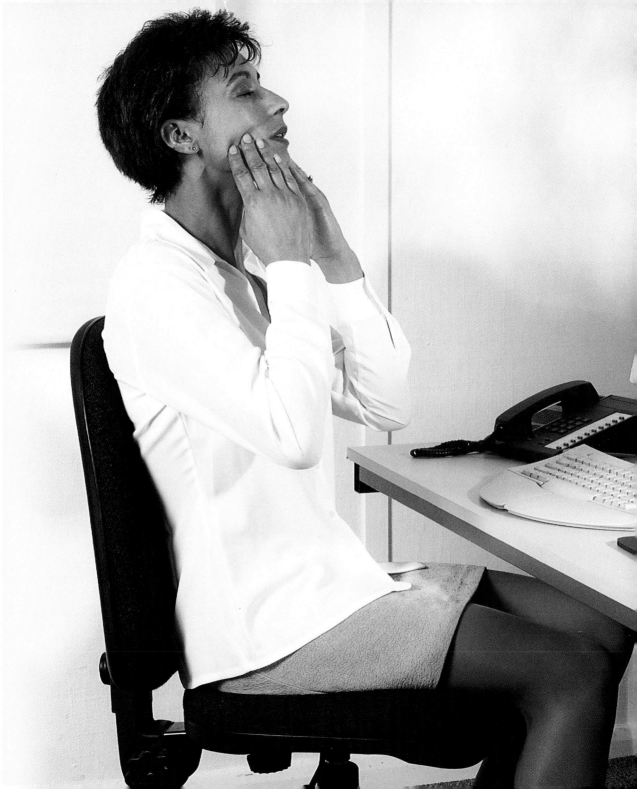

Maintaining good posture

Remain aware of your posture and physical well-being throughout your working day. Initially, this extra focus on body consciousness may feel like an effort, but with practice, it will become second nature. Once you start respecting and caring for your body as a responsive, living, breathing organism, and not a machine, it will become your greatest ally at work.

The key to good posture is to maintain balance and alignment. In particular, to prevent neck and shoulder strain, keep your neck lengthened above your shoulders and your head in a balanced position over your spine. Think of extension in terms of your spine too, carrying the image of it lengthening upwards in a relaxed manner at all times, whether you are walking, standing or sitting. Avoid slumping when sitting; instead make sure that your spine retains its natural S-shaped curves for support.

It is also vital to be conscious of your chest and shoulders, widening this area so that your lungs can expand fully as you breathe. Relax your shoulders so that they are not pulled upwards, which shortens your neck, or curled forwards, which constricts the chest. Be aware of your breathing, relaxing into your inhalation and exhalation so that you feel both your abdomen and your chest expanding and

◁ BENDING *To reach an object on the floor, sink down on your haunches, bending your knees while keeping your spine extended. Have one foot firmly placed on the ground for support and leverage. If necessary, tilt forward from your hips but keep your spine extended.*

▷ LIFTING *Pick up the object, keeping your elbows bent and arms out from your body, and draw its weight in close to your body. Using the muscles in your legs for leverage, straighten upwards from your hip joints so that your spine remains lengthened and relaxed.*

contracting under its steady inward and outward flow. Deep, relaxed breathing throughout the day is fundamental to maintaining equilibrium, especially when you are under pressure.

Lifting and bending

Common activities such as lifting and bending can cause or exacerbate back injury, largely because of the wrong use of the body when you perform such movements. To avoid strain, keep your spine straight and use the lower half of your body to dip down and straighten up. If you have an existing injury, seek help from colleagues if a heavy object needs to be moved, rather than risk making the injury worse.

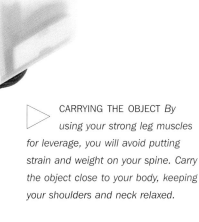

▷ CARRYING THE OBJECT *By using your strong leg muscles for leverage, you will avoid putting strain and weight on your spine. Carry the object close to your body, keeping your shoulders and neck relaxed.*

Driving in comfort

Driving a car can be very stressful, whether it is part of your occupation, or you are simply commuting to work. Prolonged periods of sitting behind the wheel, with little room to move your body, can put a lot of strain on your posture and, in particular, on the neck and shoulders. Being stuck in a traffic jam is another trigger for anxiety, which makes you tense and tighten up. Ensuring that you are as physically comfortable as possible while driving will help you to overcome these stresses.

Begin by adjusting your driving seat so that you can easily reach the pedals and steering wheel without either over-extending your arms and legs or scrunching them up. Your knees and elbows should be comfortably flexed when you have the right distance. Place your hands at a safe distance apart on the steering wheel to maintain width in your shoulders, and avoid clutching the wheel tensely. If you have a back or neck problem, purchase a back support, which attaches to the seat, or a lumbar roll, which fits snugly into the small of your back. Breathe deeply and in a relaxed way whenever you are faced with a traffic dilemma. Consciously let go of the tension. There is no point in becoming angry or impatient as this only causes your muscles to tighten. On long-

distance journeys, take regular breaks to refresh your mind, and stretch your legs to boost your blood circulation. Repeat the neck and shoulder stretches shown on pages 37–8 to release the tension from this area.

Check your posture frequently when driving and extend your neck while relaxing and widening your shoulders. Loosen your jaw and mouth and breathe deeply.

The build-up of stress while driving can cause you to grip the steering wheel too tightly. Relax your hands and allow your wrists, elbows and shoulder joints to remain at ease.

It is important to maintain the natural curvature of your spine while driving. Avoid slumping or sitting too rigidly. Invest in a good lumbar support for your driving seat.

▷ RELAXED DRIVING *Relax your shoulders at all times. Hold your head in an upright, balanced position with your neck extended but drop your chin slightly to reduce strain in the back of your neck.*

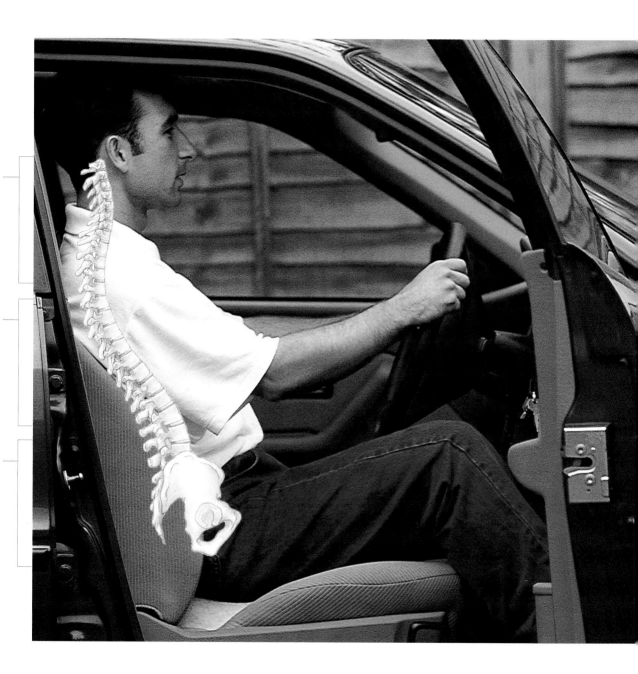

Good working posture

Our bodies are not designed for prolonged periods of sitting, so being confined to a desk for many hours a day can lead to muscular tension, especially in the lower and upper back. If your work requires you to be mostly sitting down, then take special precautions to arrange your equipment so that minimum strain is placed on your body. Aim to sit comfortably so that your spine is erect but retains its S-curves, your shoulders are relaxed, your neck is elongated and your head remains, as much as possible, in a balanced position over your spine. A specially designed office chair should be supportive to your spine and adjustable so that you can sit at the right height and angle to the work surface. The chair should rotate so there is no need to twist your body to reach objects or talk to colleagues. If your feet do not touch the floor, use a foot rest for support to the lower half of the body and to keep your knees bent.

Place equipment, such as telephone, computer monitor and keyboard, in correct positions to reduce unnecessary movements which contract or over-reach your body or make you constantly lower your head. Become aware of unconscious habits you may have developed, particularly gripping the telephone or a pen too tightly, as these may increase tension in your neck and shoulders. Make body checks so that you notice which areas are tightening up, and then relax those parts with gentle movement, exercise and self-massage. Try to vary your work so you have frequent breaks from your desk. If you are looking at a computer monitor for long periods, rest and exercise your eyes at regular intervals by changing your gaze to focus on a more distant object.

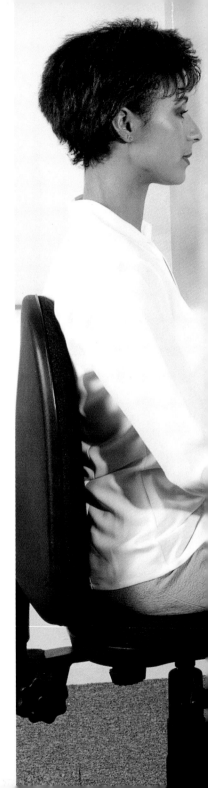

Work station

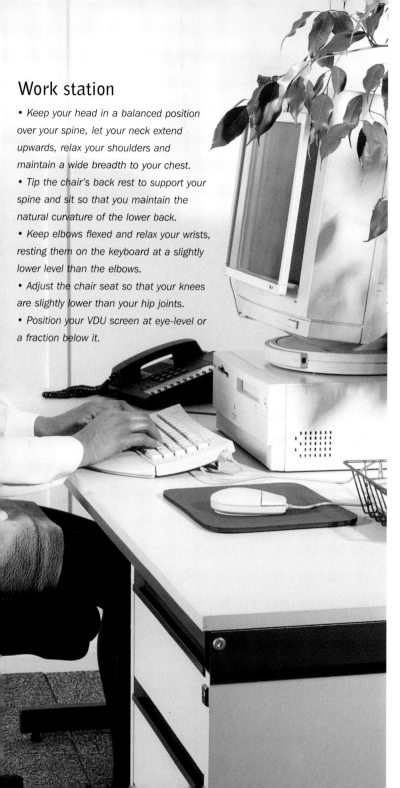

- Keep your head in a balanced position over your spine, let your neck extend upwards, relax your shoulders and maintain a wide breadth to your chest.
- Tip the chair's back rest to support your spine and sit so that you maintain the natural curvature of the lower back.
- Keep elbows flexed and relax your wrists, resting them on the keyboard at a slightly lower level than the elbows.
- Adjust the chair seat so that your knees are slightly lower than your hip joints.
- Position your VDU screen at eye-level or a fraction below it.

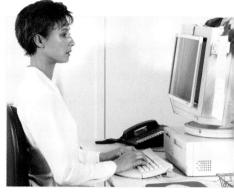

△ USE A COPY HOLDER *Constantly lowering your head will strain your neck muscles and the vertebrae at the top of the spine. Attach a copy holder to your screen so that you can easily access information.*

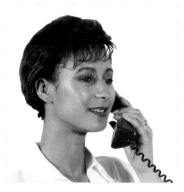

△ HOLDING THE TELEPHONE *Stay relaxed when using the telephone at work. Never hold it between your ear and shoulder as this causes considerable stress to your neck and shoulder. Avoid gripping the telephone; instead clasp it lightly.*

Exercises to release work tension

When you are concentrating on a work project, tension can creep into your body. Your breathing becomes shallow, your shoulders start to hunch up, and you may slump or strain forward in your chair. If you are aiming to meet a deadline, you are likely to work for too long without a break. While you may feel that this physical effort is helping you to accomplish your goal,

EYE EXERCISES *Prolonged staring at a computer screen causes eyestrain. Exercise your eyes regularly, rolling them in full circles five times to the right and five times to left.*

you are, in fact, draining your resources. You need to stay vigilant of your well-being and comfort while working to achieve the best results in the long-term. So, work hard but take short breaks during which you exercise and relax tense areas of your body, and take time to calm down in your mind. You will be rewarded by enjoying your work more, and keeping your energy levels higher throughout the day.

Head rotations

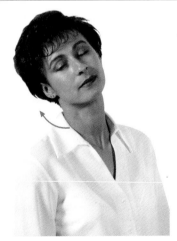

1 This head rolling exercise stretches tight neck muscles. Ensure the gentle movement originates from the vertebrae at the top of the spine. Drop your head forward and roll it slowly to your right side.

2 Let the head drop gently backwards before it rolls towards the left side of the body. Rotate the head five times to the left and repeat the exercise by rolling the head five times to the right.

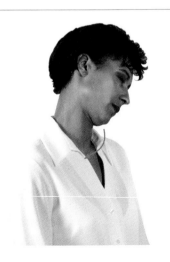

Stretching your back and chest

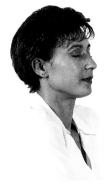

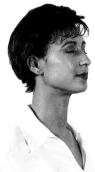

1 Relax tension in the upper body by consciously increasing and releasing it. Dangling your arms loosely, curl your shoulders forward and hold for a count of five. Then relax them back to a balanced position.

2 Now brace your shoulders backwards and hold to a count of five. Then relax them to a balanced position. This movement contracts the muscles between the shoulder blades while stretching and expanding the upper chest muscles.

BREATHE AND RELAX *Take a few minutes to completely clear your mind and restore a sense of equilibrium and peace within yourself. Sitting with your spine extended, rest your hands on your lap and close your eyes. Visualize a stream of light flowing upwards through your spine, lifting your whole being up. Breathe deeply and in a relaxed manner, focusing only on your inhalation and exhalation. Consciously let go of any stressful thoughts.*

Staying flexible

Here are some more exercises to practise throughout the day. These stretches focus mostly on releasing tension from the shoulders, arms and hands to keep the joints loose and mobile for increased flexibility in the upper body. When the upper body remains relaxed and without stress, you are naturally able to breathe more deeply and freely throughout the day. This will help you to maintain both physical and mental vitality.

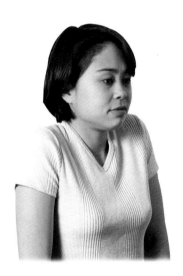

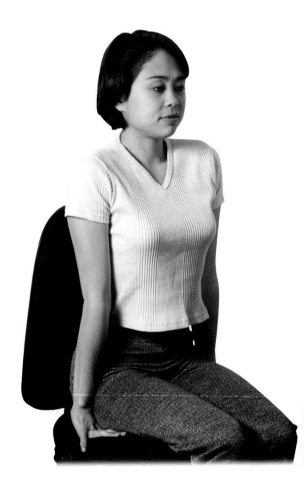

△ SHOULDER ROTATIONS *Shoulder-joint rotations can be done easily at your desk. With your arms relaxed beside your body, circle your shoulder joints backwards five times and then forwards five times. Add any of the neck stretches described on pages 50–51 to these movements.*

▷ LIFTING UPWARDS *Reverse any slumping in your back by pressing your hands against the seat of your chair to stretch and elevate your body upwards. Then gently release the stretch to settle back in your seat.*

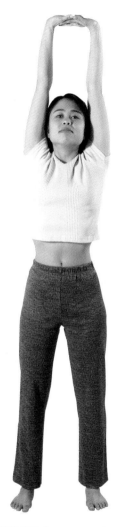

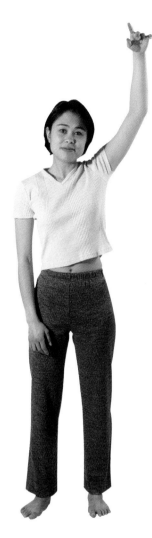

ARM SHAKE *Shake out tension from both arms, rhythmically rocking one limb at a time. Dangle the arm and let the shaking start from the fingertips so that the motion works upwards to encompass the hand, wrist, forearm, elbow, upper arm and finally the shoulder joint. This will result in the arm feeling vibrant, lengthened and relaxed.*

STRETCHING UPWARDS *Stand to stretch your whole body. Raise your arms above your head and softly interlace your fingers. Push your palms in the direction of the ceiling. Then slowly relax the pose.*

ARM CIRCLES *Loosen your shoulder girdle by making arm circles. Rotate one arm at a time, with elbows flexed and shoulders relaxed, to make five full backward circles, and five forward circles.*

Relaxing your hands

Your hands are one of the most overworked parts of your body due to their actions of repetitive movements, gripping and overstretching. Stop to relax them every now and again to reduce a build-up of strain in the joints, tendons and the many small bones. By contracting and extending your hands frequently, you can reverse the harmful effects caused by the constant repetition of one type of movement and reduce the risk of long-term injury.

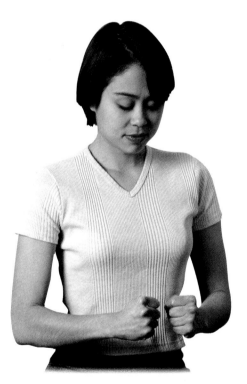

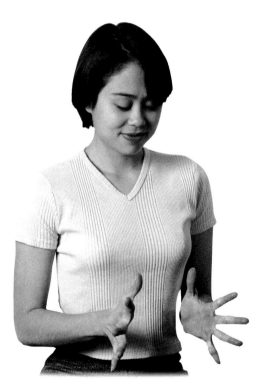

1 *Make tight fists of your hands to contract their muscles and tendons. Hold this position for a count of five. Do this and the next exercise three times.*

2 *Open up your hands to extend your fingers as far as possible and to stretch the tendons. Hold this stretch for a count of five before relaxing your hands.*

Supple Hands

The hands, like the feet, have reflex points which correspond to internal organs. By stimulating these reflex points, you can invigorate and relax the internal structures of your physiological system. In addition, the thousands of nerve endings in your hands transmit vital sensory information to your brain about the external world. Keeping your hands relaxed and free from tension is therefore important to your overall vitality and sensory awardness.

3 Finally, with your elbows bent and at right angles to your body, place your hands in the prayer gesture in front of your chest. Separate the heels slightly to press the fingers and upper palms together for an expanding stretch.

Self-massage at work

Just a few minutes of self-massage is all it takes to revive your mental alertness and undo the physical stress that can accumulate during a concentrated period of work. Stop for short breaks regularly throughout the day, or whenever you are feeling particularly stressed, and apply these simple strokes to relieve stress and restore energy. They will leave you feeling more alert and able to cope with a tough work situation. These following steps of self-massage zone in on key tension points in the upper body that are prone to gather strain while you are working at a desk. They focus particularly on the head, face, neck and shoulder area. For the best results, spend approximately one minute on each step.

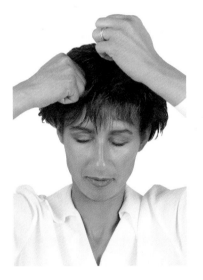

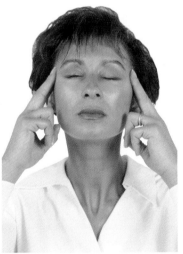

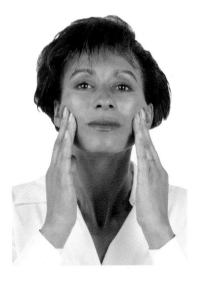

△ REVIVING YOUR MIND *With your fists close to each other, lightly pummel them all over the surface of your head in a bouncing and rhythmic motion. Keep your fists loose and your wrists relaxed. This movement boosts circulation to your scalp.*

△ SOOTHING YOUR TEMPLES *Release strain from your eyes and brow with backward circular strokes applied to your temples from the first two fingertips of each hand. Close your eyes and soothe away tension with backward-flowing motions.*

△ MASSAGING YOUR CHEEKS *Relax your cheeks and mouth with backward-flowing circular motions applied from your fingertips. Ensure the cheek muscles move beneath the spiralling touch of your fingers, so that your mouth loosens up.*

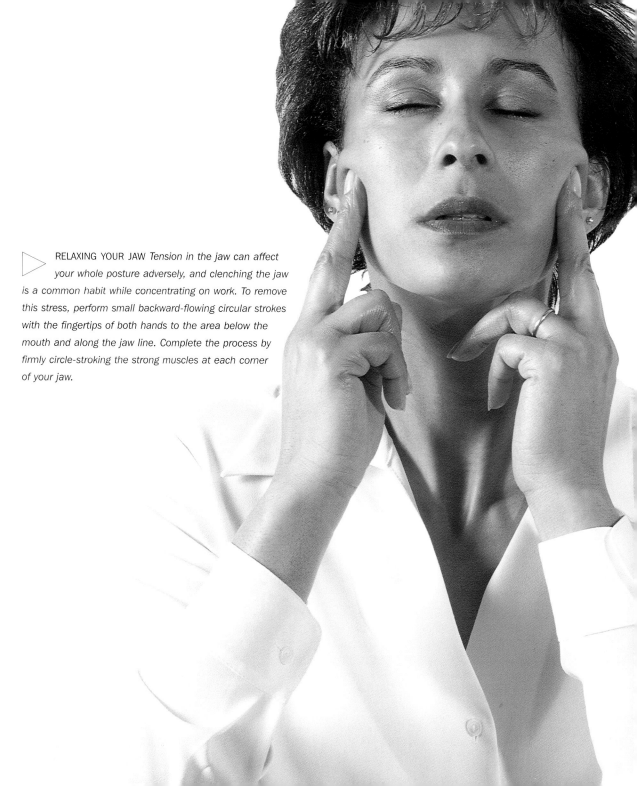

▷ RELAXING YOUR JAW *Tension in the jaw can affect your whole posture adversely, and clenching the jaw is a common habit while concentrating on work. To remove this stress, perform small backward-flowing circular strokes with the fingertips of both hands to the area below the mouth and along the jaw line. Complete the process by firmly circle-stroking the strong muscles at each corner of your jaw.*

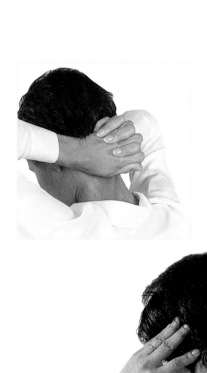

KNEADING YOUR NECK *Placing your hands behind your neck, softly lock your fingers together so that the neck is nestled between your hands. Press the heels firmly into the flesh, scooping and squeezing it as they slide towards each other. Work this kneading motion up and down the back of the neck.*

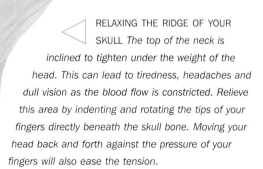

RELAXING THE RIDGE OF YOUR SKULL *The top of the neck is inclined to tighten under the weight of the head. This can lead to tiredness, headaches and dull vision as the blood flow is constricted. Relieve this area by indenting and rotating the tips of your fingers directly beneath the skull bone. Moving your head back and forth against the pressure of your fingers will also ease the tension.*

Using a massage tool

A massage tool can be used to make circular motions out across the top of your chest towards the shoulders to release tension from contracted pectoral muscles which may constrict your breathing. Make circular motions out and across, releasing your upper chest (see right). Circulate the pegs over one side of the body at a time, moving from the centre of your chest towards the shoulder joint. Lighten the pressure when rotating the massager over bone.

Rotate your massage tool over the top of your arm to bring relief to tight muscles (see left). Continue circulating the pegs down the lower half of the limb, on to the back of your hand and then over your palm. Then repeat these strokes on the other arm.

▷ STRETCHING YOUR FINGERS *Stretch and stimulate each finger to release stiffness. Grasp the little finger of one hand between the forefinger and thumb of the other hand. Gently pull along the length of the finger, giving the tip a little squeeze before snapping your fingers away from it. Return to the original hold and squeeze gently up along the whole finger. Apply these motions to the other fingers and thumb and then repeat them on the other hand.*

Quick-fixes for colleagues

Encourage your colleagues to learn the basic massage techniques described in this book and to become adept at using the massage tool. This should be an easy task once they realize how speedily relief from tension can be obtained from these 'quick-fix' remedial techniques. Then you can respond to one another in times of stress, by applying the strokes during work breaks to restore an overall sense of relaxation.

The massage treatments shown in this chapter are appropriate for the more formal atmosphere of the office environment, as they can be applied to someone who is fully clothed and who remains seated. Keep a massage tool in the office so it is always available when needed. Use it in conjunction with other strokes, or on its own for colleagues who prefer mechanical rather than manual contact.

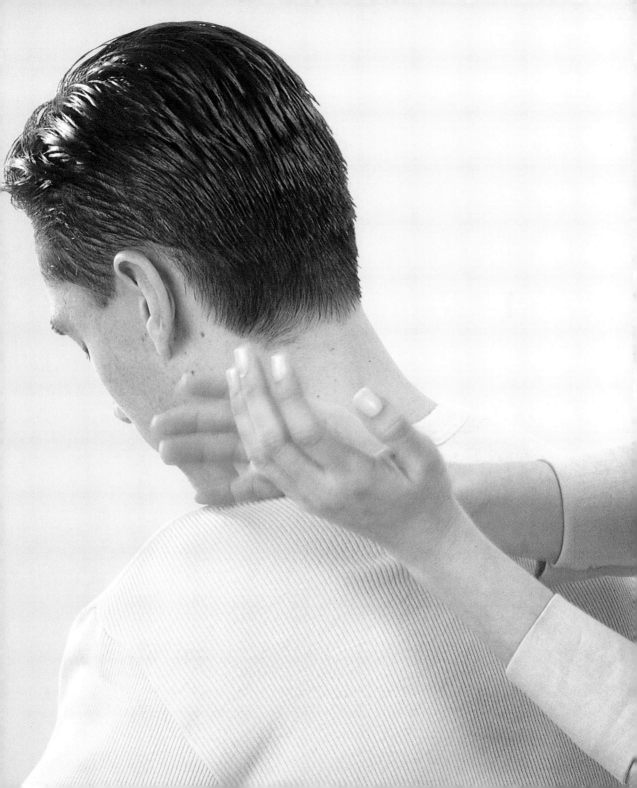

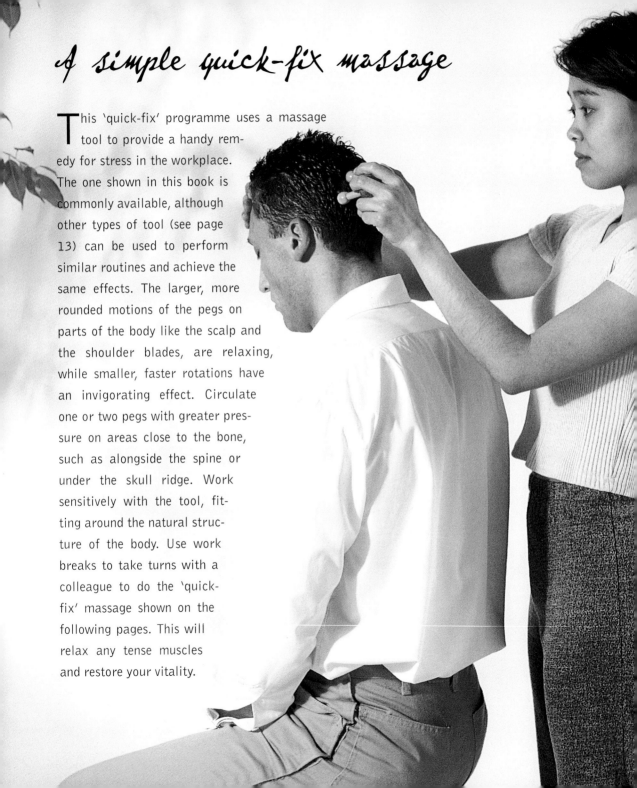

A simple quick-fix massage

This 'quick-fix' programme uses a massage tool to provide a handy remedy for stress in the workplace. The one shown in this book is commonly available, although other types of tool (see page 13) can be used to perform similar routines and achieve the same effects. The larger, more rounded motions of the pegs on parts of the body like the scalp and the shoulder blades, are relaxing, while smaller, faster rotations have an invigorating effect. Circulate one or two pegs with greater pressure on areas close to the bone, such as alongside the spine or under the skull ridge. Work sensitively with the tool, fitting around the natural structure of the body. Use work breaks to take turns with a colleague to do the 'quick-fix' massage shown on the following pages. This will relax any tense muscles and restore your vitality.

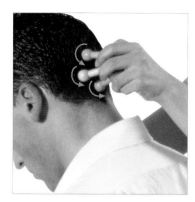

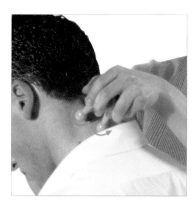

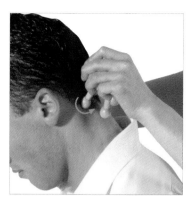

△ SCALP *Supporting your colleague's forehead in the palm of one hand, use the other hand to circulate the massager at an even pressure on the scalp so that the whole of the head is stimulated.*

△ NECK *Being very gentle, depress the pegs onto the back of the neck, making small, flowing circles to loosen and manipulate the muscles.*

△ UNDER SKULL RIDGE *Tilt the massage tool so that you can rotate a single peg on one place at a time along the area directly beneath the ridge of the skull. Work in towards the spine on both sides.*

▷ SPINE *With one hand supporting the shoulder, tip the massager inwards so that two pegs indent into the muscle directly beside the spine. Rotate the pegs on one area at a time, working from the shoulder blades to the top of the back.*

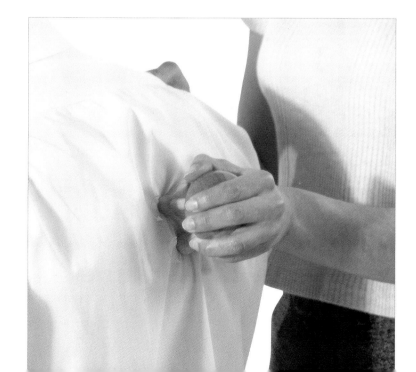

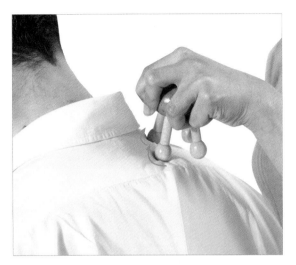

Along the spine

Strokes applied to the spine and those described here should be applied first to one side of the body and then to the other.

◁ BASE OF NECK *Relieve tension from the area surrounding the base of the neck by rotating the front two pegs of the massage tool into the muscles, deepening the pressure as they loosen up.*

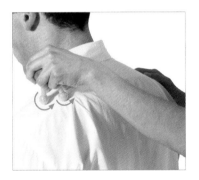

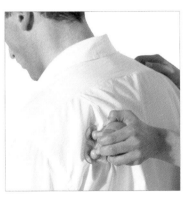

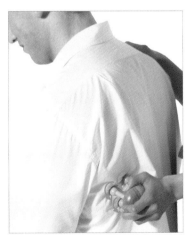

△ TOP OF SHOULDERS *Relax the top of the shoulder with smooth, flowing circular strokes. Use an even pressure with the four pegs and work from the neck towards the shoulder joint. Decrease the pressure as you massage over the bone.*

△ SHOULDER BLADES *Continue the smooth, rounded motions firmly onto the muscle that covers the flat, triangular bone of the shoulder blade, easing away tightness and tension and increasing flexibility.*

△ RIBCAGE *Slide the tool over to the side of the ribcage, circulating the pegs along the edge and base of the shoulder blade to boost circulation to the tissues.*

▽ TOPS OF ARMS *Apply small, vigorous rotations over the muscles at the top of the arm to increase flexibility in the whole limb and ease the shoulder girdle. Repeat all the appropriate strokes on the other side of the body.*

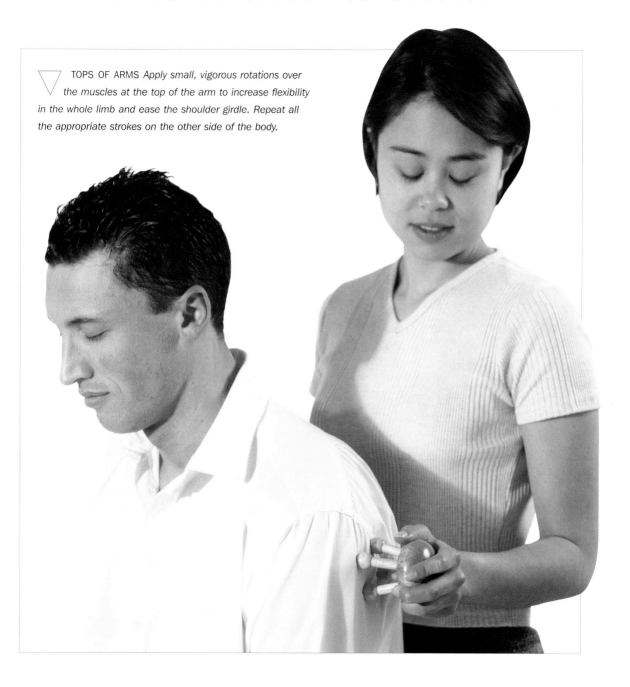

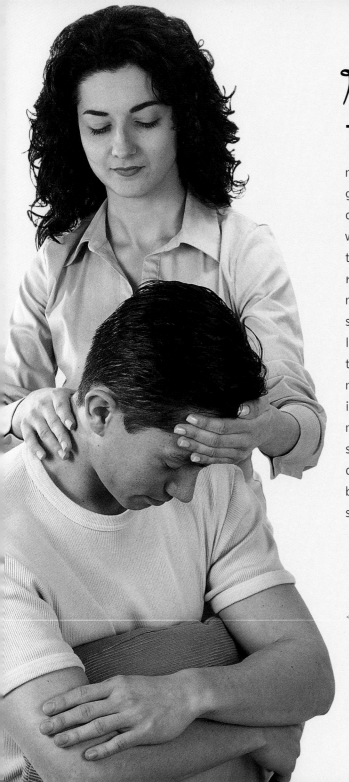

Ten-minute massage

The tactile contact of hands on the body adds an effective dimension to a 'quick-fix' treatment. Using your hands, you can perform a great variety of massage techniques which thoroughly relax and invigorate the muscles. The warm and soothing quality of this massage, even through clothes, also induces greater overall relaxation. The techniques that form this ten-minute massage are adapted from the basic strokes described on pages 16–31. Refer back to learn how to perform them, and to understand their effects and benefits. In the office environment where strokes are applied over clothing, it is not possible to recreate the same sliding motions of a massage using oil, but you can construct a programme that is close to it. Ask your colleague to straddle a chair so as to face its back. Place a cushion in front of their chest for support under the pressure of the strokes.

◁ HEAD HOLD *Begin with a hold that allows your colleague some moments to relax. Place one hand gently over his forehead and rest the other against the back of his neck. Let your hands impart a calming sense of stillness.*

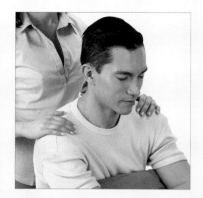

SHOULDER HOLD *Perform this hold by resting your hands gently on your colleague's shoulders. Their warmth will initiate a release of tension from the shoulder girdle as he begins to unwind.*

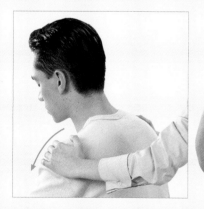

SWEEPING THE SHOULDERS *Moulding your hands to the shoulders, glide your palms out and down the top of the arms. Sweep the stroke out and away from the body.*

SWEEPING THE BACK *Rest your hands on the shoulders to either side of the neck before sweeping them down each side of the spine. Fan them out and away from the body towards the sides. Repeat twice more.*

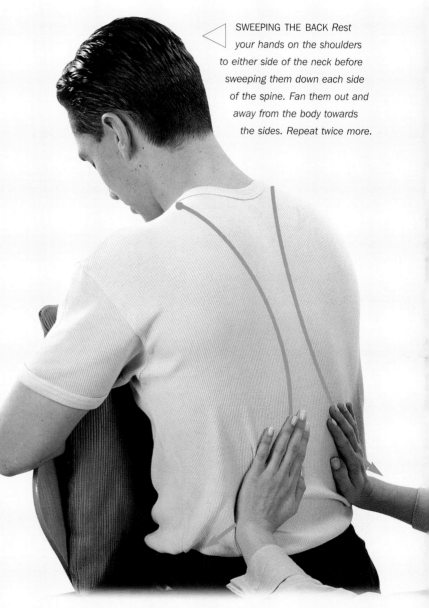

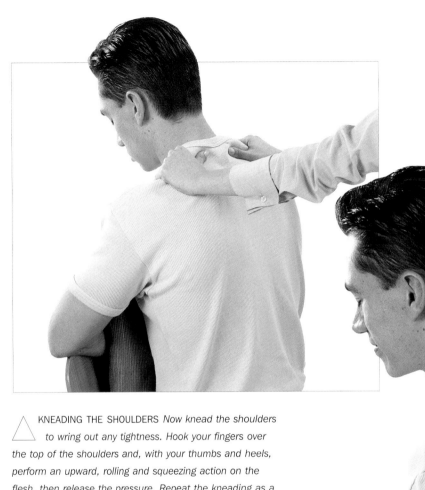

△ KNEADING THE SHOULDERS *Now knead the shoulders to wring out any tightness. Hook your fingers over the top of the shoulders and, with your thumbs and heels, perform an upward, rolling and squeezing action on the flesh, then release the pressure. Repeat the kneading as a continuous motion for at least one minute to soften up the muscles.*

▷ KNEADING THE ARMS *Mould each hand to the top of the arms. Apply pressure with your fingers and heels to make a continuous squeeze-and-release motion on the muscles, kneading down towards the elbows. Repeat the sequence twice more to loosen the arms.*

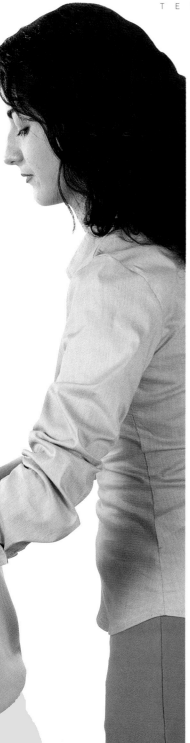

▷ KNEADING THE NECK *With the head dropped forward, interlink* your fingers *lightly and wrap your palms and heels over the top of the neck. Gently but firmly slide the heels towards each other to squeeze the underlying muscles, taking care not to pinch the skin. Release the pressure and repeat the stroke down towards the base of the neck.*

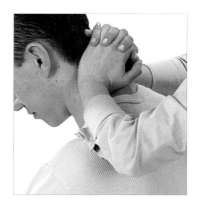

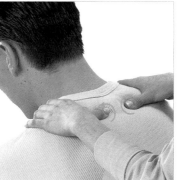

◁ RELEASING STROKES *Grind away tension from the area* surrounding the base of the neck. *Clasp your fingers over the shoulders and sink your thumbs slowly into the muscles. Circulate your thumbs on one spot at a time deepening the pressure on the first half of the circle.*

▷ DEEPER PETRISSAGE *Focus the pressure on one thumb only to* penetrate to deeper levels of tissue on *tight points along either side of the spine. Support the front of the body with one hand and slowly depress the other thumb into a tense spot before rotating it several times. Then move the thumb to the next tense area. Complete by repeating the sweeping strokes down the spine.*

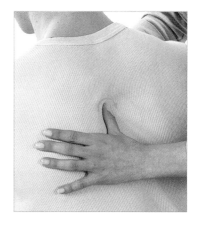

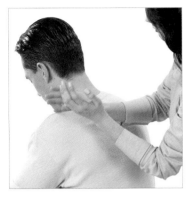

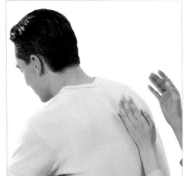

HACKING ALONG THE SPINE
Continue the hacking stroke down each side of the spine to the middle of the back, taking care not to strike directly over the vertebrae. This will stimulate tired muscles and refresh the upper body.

HACKING THE SHOULDERS
Briskly hack over the top of both shoulders to break down tightness in the muscles and to invigorate the circulation. Do not hack directly on top of bone.

PUMMELLING SHOULDERS
Pummelling can be used as an alternative to hacking, or as a follow-up, to increase the revitalizing effect of the office massage. With relaxed wrists and loose fists, pummel one hand briskly after the other over the top of the shoulders.

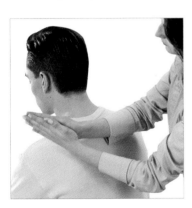

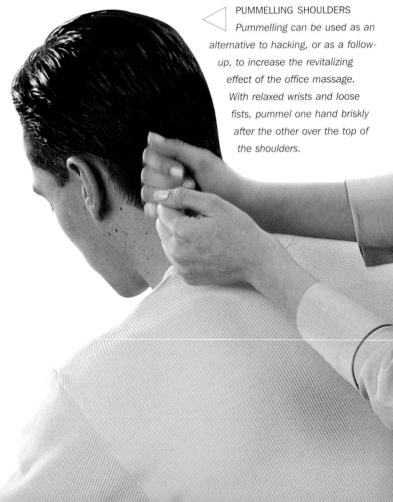

DOUBLE-HANDED HACKING
Double-handed hacking has a gentler impact on the body than the previous hacking stroke. Placing your hands together, rhythmically bounce the sides of your hands simultaneously over the top of both shoulders.

HEAD MASSAGE *A scalp massage will clear and refresh the mind. Placing your thumbs on the head* for support, make a slight claw shape with your hands and massage over the entire surface of the scalp with backward-flowing fingertip rotations.

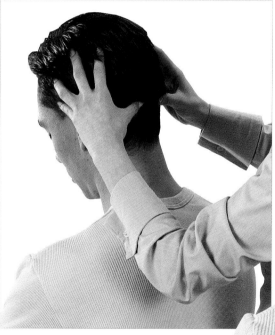

QUIET FINISH *Complete your ten-minute massage with a gentle hold.* Lay your hands softly and symmetrically on his head, focusing your attention towards this soothing contact. Then withdraw your hands slowly.

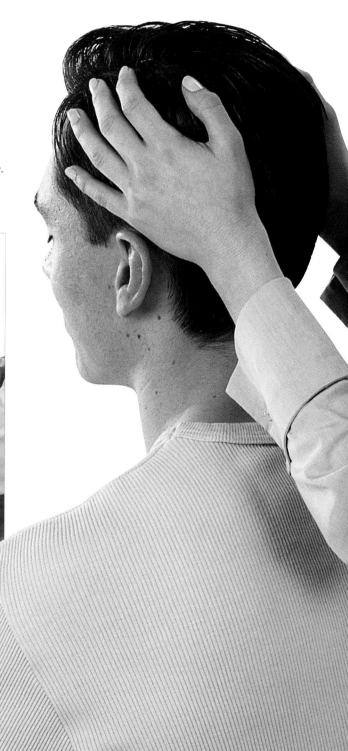

Pressure-point massage

This short session of applying sustained thumb pressure to specific points on the upper back can bring relief to a colleague who is experiencing shoulder and neck pain or a headache. The pressure-point massage works along the energy meridians of the upper body (see panel, opposite) to release deep-seated tension in the muscles. While it does not strictly follow the form of traditional Shiatsu massage, which is usually performed on floor level and adheres to specific postures, stretches and movements, the stimulation of the pressure points can free blocked energy and initiate a release of muscular tension.

Follow the points illustrated in the photographs, pressing at distances of about a thumb's-width apart. Lean your weight slowly into your thumbs and press on each point for about five seconds, before releasing the pressure gradually. Be aware that some points may feel particularly tender, so ask your colleague to warn you if the pressure becomes uncomfortable. Before doing the pressure-point massage, warm and loosen the shoulders with some kneading and percussion strokes.

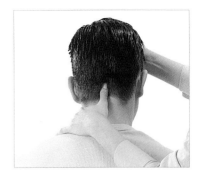

⚠ **1** TOP OF NECK *Gently probe with your thumb to locate the hollow space at the top of the spine under the skull ridge. Supporting the head with one hand, indent with the other thumb as though pressing upwards.*

Pressure points

- TOP OF NECK *Eases stiff neck, relieves headache*
- BASE OF SKULL (either side of spine) *Alleviates neck pain, clears sinuses*
- SHOULDERS *Reduces shoulder pain, relaxes shoulder girdle*
- SPINE *Relieves back pain, relaxes spine, benefits internal organs*
- SHOULDER BLADE *Helps frozen shoulder pain, relaxes shoulders, eases breathing*

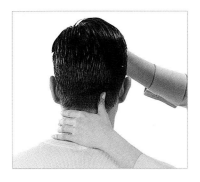

2 BASE OF SKULL *These pressure points at the base of the skull are situated about a thumb's-width from either side of the top of the neck. Working on one side at a time, depress your thumb gradually into the hollow space directly beneath the bone before releasing the pressure slowly.*

3 SHOULDERS *Lean your weight into your thumbs to press them along the top of the shoulders, moving from the base of the neck to the outer edge of the shoulders. Apply pressure at gaps of one thumb's width.*

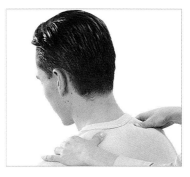

4 SPINE *Press your thumbs into the channel either side of the vertebrae, from shoulders level down to the base of the shoulder blades. Shift your weight to and fro to apply and release the pressure.*

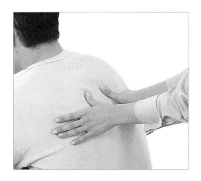

5 SHOULDER BLADES *Find the slight indentation at the centre of the shoulder bone. Place one hand at the front of the shoulder to support the body, and press steadily but gently into this point with the other thumb. Repeat on the other shoulder blade.*

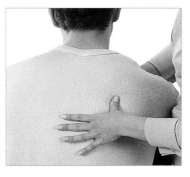

Energy meridians

Traditional Eastern healing arts, such as Shiatsu, acupressure and acupuncture, are now widely accepted for the prevention and treatment of many physical disorders, including back problems and neck and shoulder pain. These alternative health therapies work on the premise that within the body there are pathways, known as meridians, through which the force of life energy flows. If this natural stream becomes sluggish or blocked, the overall health of the body is upset.

It is believed that certain locations along the meridians act as key energy points which can be stimulated to release the energy flow and restore the body's own healing processes.

CHAPTER FIVE

Passive movements

Releasing tension is as much a psychological response as a physical one, especially if you feel under pressure to stay in control all the time. If you can relate to such phrases as 'carrying the world on your shoulders' or 'being up to your neck in it', then the passive movements described in this chapter may help you let go of both mental and physical stress. These techniques, which here are focused on the neck and shoulder area, unlock the tension and contraction around major segments and joints of the body.

The session consists of passive movements designed to encourage you to allow the active partner to lift and take the weight of a body part, such as the head or an arm, and to move it gently without your assistance. The ability to release control of this weight and movement into your partner's hands enables you to relax deeply. Practise the passive movements with a partner or a friend in the comfort of your home, where it is easier to relinquish the need to be always in charge.

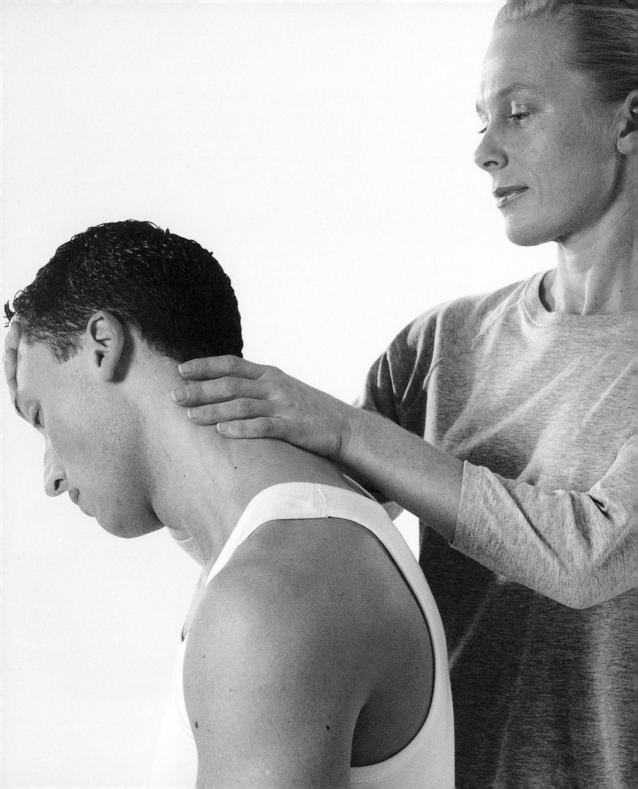

Confident hands

Passive movements need practice to be effective. The person executing them must learn to impart a feeling of confidence through their hands as they make the gentle but persuasive movements on the other person's body. This allows the recipient to feel secure enough to give up control and to remain passive and trusting while his partner is moving his body.

The head, neck, shoulder joints and arms should be moved slowly according to their natural motion so no force is applied. Never push a part of the body beyond its point of resistance. However, relaxation in an area of tension can be encouraged by focusing the movement on the point just below the threshold of resistance. The person receiving the treatment should breathe comfortably but deeply, focusing his attention on the motion while releasing the weight of the body part into his partner's hands

and giving up any attempt to aid the movements. This mental and physical letting-go initiates a deep release of tension in contracted areas.

Head roll

The rolling motion of the head increases suppleness in the neck and upper spine so that the head feels freer and lighter. The person receiving should sit, with spine relaxed yet extended, on a chair or stool. Using gentle pressure from the forehand, circulate the head three times to the left and then the right.

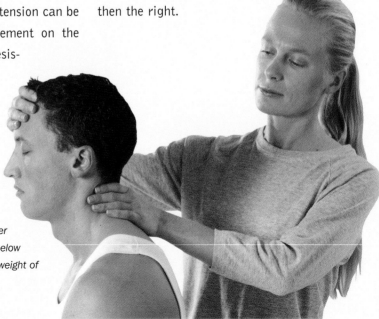

▷ *Place one hand softly on your partner's forehead and rest the other supportively on the back of his neck, just below the base of the skull. Ask him to drop the weight of his head into your hand.*

Lifting shoulders

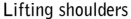

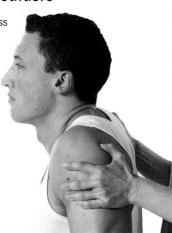

This passive movement releases stiffness in the neck by first exacerbating the upward-holding pattern and then lowering the shoulders slowly so they drop back to a relaxed level. Clasp the top of each arm with your hands, then lever them upwards, raising your partner's shoulders. Encourage him to take a deep inhalation of breath as you do so. As he exhales, lower the weight of the arms and shoulders back down. Repeat the movement twice more.

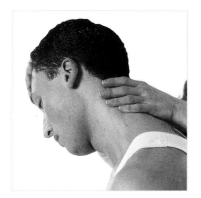

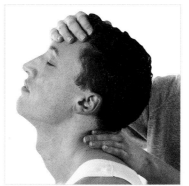

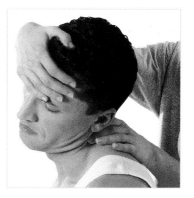

/2\ *Begin to circulate your partner's head slowly to the right to create a stretch in the left side of his neck. Ensure that the origin of the movement comes from the vertebra at the top of the spine.*

/3\ *Continue to slowly roll the head around so that its weight drops back, creating a flexion at the top of the spine. Whenever you feel your partner is trying to assist the motion, encourage him to give you the weight and movement of his head.*

/4\ *As the head continues its rotation to the left side, the right side of the neck is stretched. Roll the head back to a central, balanced position before repeating the motion.*

Head and neck movements

The passive movements described here focus on the head and neck. The aim of the movements is to encourage your partner to give up the heavy weight of their head into your hands, enabling you to lift it up and then lower it back down. This is followed by a movement that turns the head from side to side. Many people find it difficult to release control of the weight and movement of the head. The head represents the mind, or 'master', over feelings. In times of stress, tension forms in the shoulders to cut off from uncomfortable emotions. To that person, letting go in this area may feel like relinquishing mental control, so it is important that your hands feel confident and reassuring and that the motions used are slow and steady.

Before starting the movements, the passive partner (the person receiving the massage) should lie comfortably on a rug or mattress on the floor. Their partner should encourage them to take some deep breaths and make them feel completely relaxed and comfortable.

If you are doing the massage, position yourself behind your partner's head. Take care of your own posture before and during the movements, keeping your spine and neck lengthened and your shoulders widened. When working on ground level, kneel so that one knee is flexed with the foot placed on the floor. This enables you to lever yourself upwards using the lower half of your body, and avoids placing strain on your own spine.

Head turning

This passive movement slightly lifts and turns the head from side to side to stretch and relax the neck and the muscle attachments under the base of the skull. Repeat the two steps to turn the head three times to each side.

Head lift and lower

With this passive movement the person giving the massage lifts the head to stretch the neck. Pause after each movement so that your partner can savour its releasing effects.

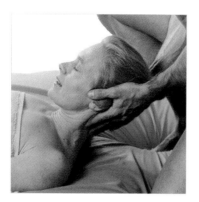

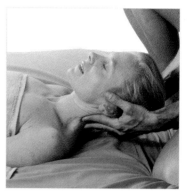

◁ **I** *Slide your hands behind your partner's head, fingers pointed downwards on the back of her neck with her head nestled safely in your palms. Place your thumbs beside each ear. Now follow steps 2 and 3. Repeat three times.*

△ **2** *Lever yourself upwards carefully as you raise your partner's head to bring a good stretch to the back of the neck. Ensure that the head remains in line with the spine throughout the movement.*

△ **3** *Sink back on your haunches as you slowly and steadily lower her head down to the ground, keeping your hands securely in position. Repeat twice more.*

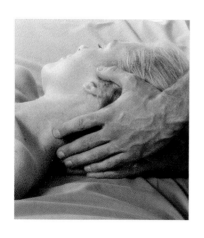

◁ **I** *Keeping your hands securely in the same position as before (above), lift the head a couple of centimetres off the floor. Roll it slowly to the right so that the side of the face is cradled in your right hand.*

▷ **2** *Now smoothly roll the head to the left so that it rests against your left hand. Then return the head to a balanced position in line with the spine.*

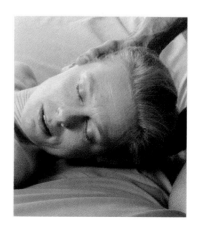

Shoulder movements

Let your hands convey, through the movements shown here, the important feeling of width to the chest and shoulders, and length to the arms, so that your partner is able to release tension from constricted areas in the upper body. For the first step, remain in the position behind the head described on pages 78–9, and then move to the side of the body to complete the techniques. Work first on one side of the body and then the other. At the end of this session, your partner should feel a sense of expansion in the chest.

1 PRESSING THE SHOULDERS *Place your hands over your partner's shoulders, so that the fingers rest on the top of the chest while your palms cup over the joints. Steadily lean your weight into your hands to gently press the shoulders back towards the mattress so that the chest expands. Then slowly release the pressure. Do this movement three times.*

2 WIDENING THE SHOULDER *Raise the back of the shoulder slightly with your left hand, then transfer to your right hand. Gently move your left hand, palm upwards with fingers towards spine, to rest beneath the shoulder blade. Place your right hand over the parallel area on the front of the body. Pause to allow your partner to relax her shoulder cradled between your hands, before slowly drawing out both hands to the edge of the shoulder, bringing a release to this area.*

Lengthening the arm

For this movement, you need to reposition yourself to kneel beside your partner's hip, so you are facing the top of her shoulder. The movement creates a relaxing stretch that brings a feeling of length and release to the whole limb. Glide your hands down her arm in a smooth and steady fashion.

1 Cup your hands lightly over the shoulder joint, placing the left hand on top and the right hand below. Ensuring that the elbow stays slightly flexed, gently but firmly slide your hands down both sides of the arm to just below the elbow joint.

2 Lean back to continue gliding your hands down the lower arm towards the wrist. Lightly grip the wrist with your left hand, while sliding your right hand further down to clasp the hand. Lean a little further backwards to exert a very gentle pull on the shoulder joint, to create a relaxing stretch.

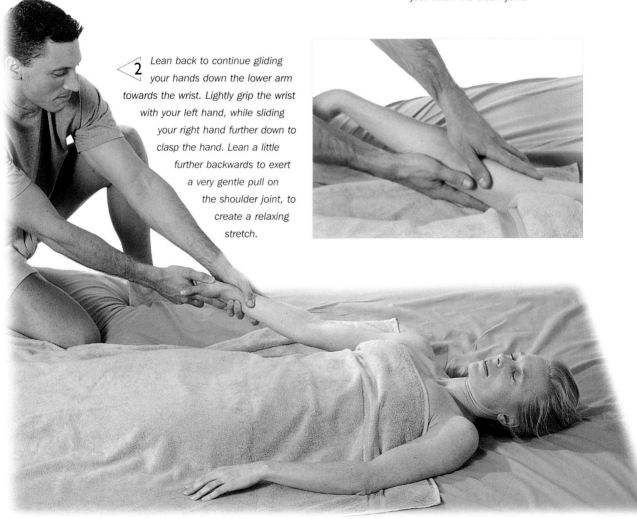

Passive movements on the arms

These passive movements on the arm can increase flexibility and relaxation in the limb and shoulder joint. You are aiming to release tension from the shoulder by taking the weight of the arm, lifting and lowering it, and then moving it so that the motions come from the ball-and-socket structure of the shoulder joint. Pause briefly if you feel that your partner is trying to aid the movements, or if the arm stiffens, so that she becomes aware of the resistance, and then continue. Gently persuading your partner to relax is fine, but never try to pressure her, either through words or movements, into releasing tension, as this is counterproductive. If your partner is unable to let go of her tension on this occasion, work within the parameters of the resistance, as this can still initiate a degree of relaxation.

◁ LIFTING THE ARM *Position yourself beside your partner's shoulder. Clasp her wrist with your left hand and support the back of her elbow with your right hand. With the elbow joint relaxed, slowly lift and lower the upper arm several times. Then gently rock the arm towards and away from the body several times.*

▷ STRETCHING THE ARM *Lever yourself slowly upwards to raise and stretch the arm so that the movement exerts a very gentle pull on the shoulder joint. Release this stretch by steadily lowering the arm down again, supporting the back of the elbow with one hand as it bends.*

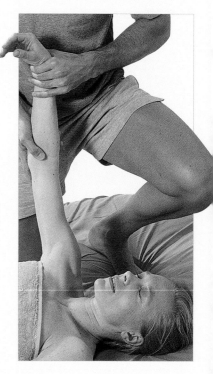

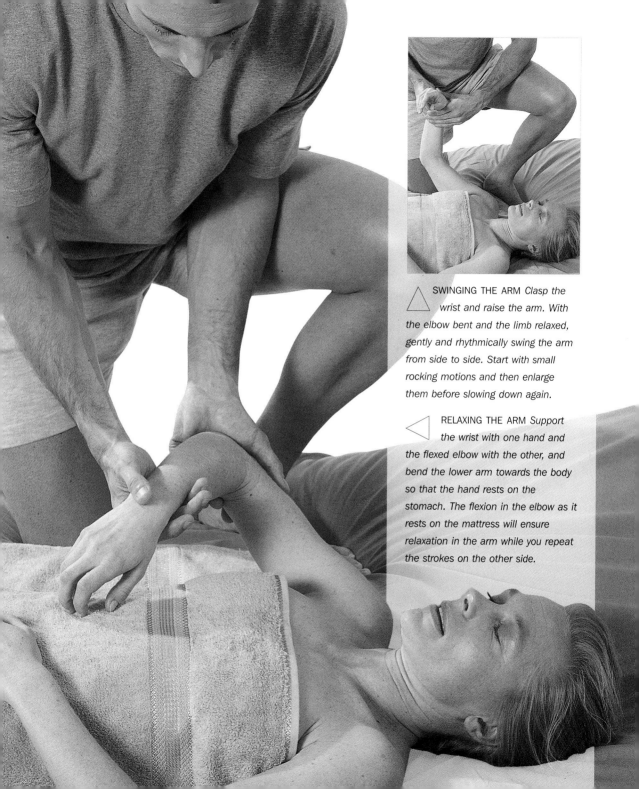

△ SWINGING THE ARM *Clasp the wrist and raise the arm.* With the elbow bent and the limb relaxed, gently and rhythmically swing the arm from side to side. Start with small rocking motions and then enlarge them before slowing down again.

◁ RELAXING THE ARM *Support the wrist with one hand and* the flexed elbow with the other, and bend the lower arm towards the body so that the hand rests on the stomach. The flexion in the elbow as it rests on the mattress will ensure relaxation in the arm while you repeat the strokes on the other side.

A head, neck and face massage

Let your home be the place where you unwind after a stressful day at work. In this environment, you can enjoy the luxury of receiving a pampering head, face and neck massage, knowing that you can now relax. The strokes shown in this chapter combine to create a massage that is soothing and calming to the mind, while at the same time removing physical tension and discomfort. A head, neck and face massage can leave you feeling refreshed and free to enjoy the rest of your evening. It can also be an invaluable aid to help you relax sufficiently to enjoy a good night's sleep.

Share the pleasure of giving or receiving this massage with a partner or close friend. Ensure the room is warm and comfortable, and that the lighting is low. To create a peaceful ambience, try massaging by candlelight and play soothing or meditative music in the background. Rub a small amount of lotion or oil into your hands to ensure the strokes move smoothly over the skin.

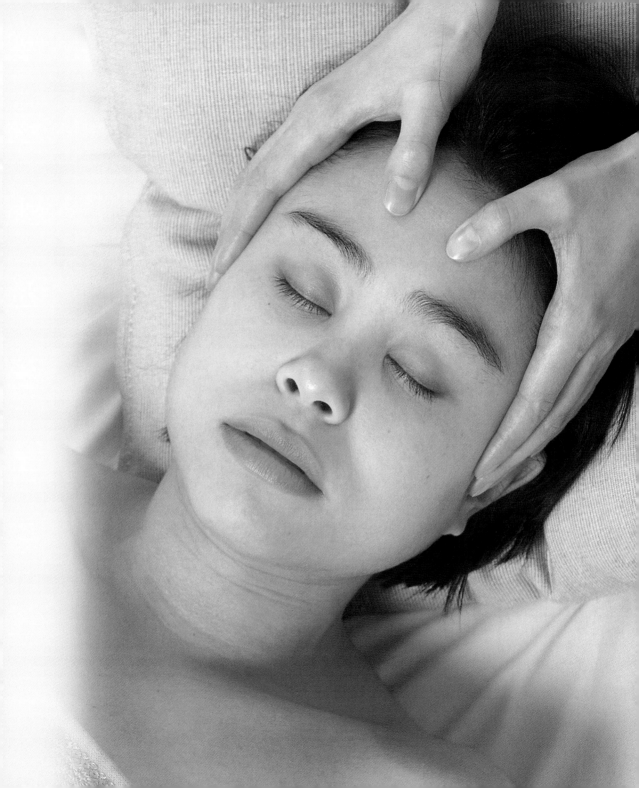

A connecting stroke

This stroke encompasses the upper chest, shoulders, neck and head in one long sweeping movement. It creates a sense of connection between the head and the body, bringing width to the shoulders and length to the neck. The movement of your hands should be firm, confident and steady as you apply varying degrees of pressure at different stages of the stroke. Be flexible in your wrists so that your hands can easily slide around the shoulders and turn to glide under the neck. To perform the stroke, kneel or sit behind your friend's head. Perform the stroke three times.

▽ **HANDS ON CHEST** *Start the stroke by laying both hands flat over the centre of the chest, at the top of the breastbone. Rest them here for some moments as your massage partner relaxes and deepens her breathing.*

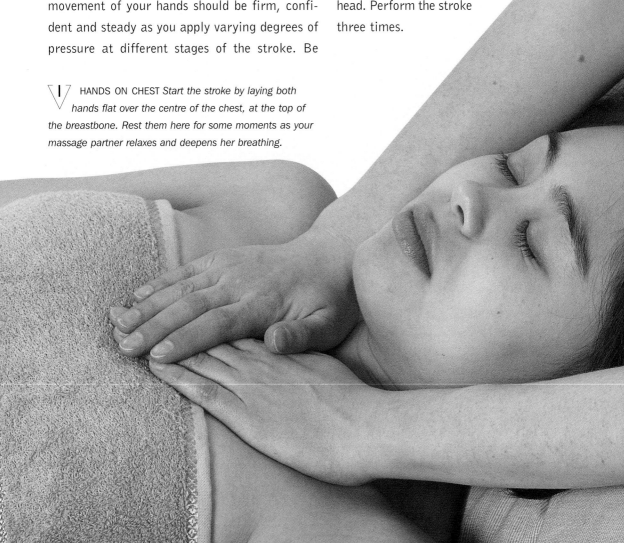

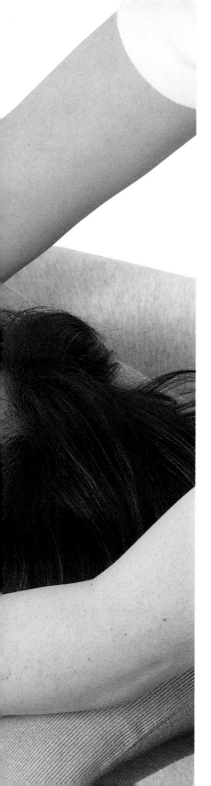

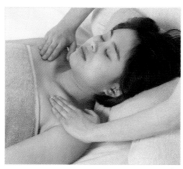

2 **WIDENING THE CHEST** *Glide your hands upwards and then* turn them to draw them out across the top of the chest, towards the edges of the shoulders. As you do this, increase the pressure to create a releasing stretch and to bring width to the upper chest.

3 **ENCIRCLING THE SHOULDERS** *Flex your wrists and decrease* the pressure in your hands as they encircle the joints to glide lightly up the back of the shoulder muscles towards the base of the neck.

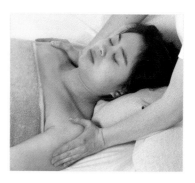

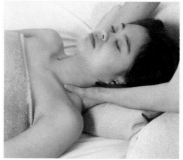

4 **BASE OF NECK** *Straighten your wrists to manoeuvre your* fingers under the back, so that they point down on each side of the top of the spine, while the back of the neck rests comfortably in your palms.

5 **NECK STRETCH** *Steadily pull your hands up the back of the* neck, gliding your thumbs behind the ears, so that the neck is gently stretched and lengthened. Lift the head slightly to slide your hands behind it and out of the body.

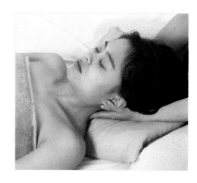

Relaxing strokes for the head and neck

Follow up the relaxing connection stroke (see pages 86–7) by focusing the massage on the neck, applying a stroke which stretches and releases tension from the muscles that turn and move the head back and forth. A neck massage can do much more than relieve stiffness from the immediate muscle group, because once this area becomes supple the posture and structure of the whole body begins to relax. The neck is the bridge between the head and the body, and is, therefore, the area that links our mental and physical processes. By having the strains that accumulate in the neck and shoulder region alleviated, the person receiving the massage not only feels relaxed, but begins to feel more whole and integrated.

Releasing neck tension

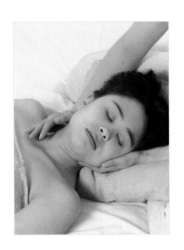

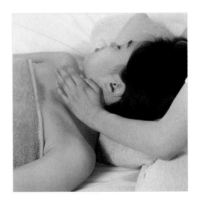

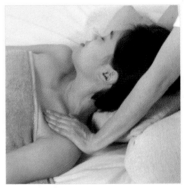

△ ANCHORING THE HEAD *To steady the head for the following strokes, turn it to nestle in the passive palm. Curl the last two fingers of that hand slightly under the neck to secure the position of the head.*

△ 1 *Fit the heel of your hand to the side of the neck, placing it just below the base of the skull. The rest of your hand should be slightly raised and flexed. Firmly but sensitively slide the heel down to the base of the neck.*

△ 2 *Flatten your fingers out to the base of the neck, so that the shoulder is encompassed by the palm and heel. As you slide your hand towards the edge of the shoulder, increase the pressure of your stroke, gently pressing the shoulder joint downwards.*

In this stroke, your hand should shape itself to the contours of the neck and shoulders. All parts of your hand are used during this stroke, starting with pressure from the heel, then the palm, and finally the upward glide of your fingers. It is performed as one long flowing motion and should be applied three times in succession to one side of the neck. This is followed by a scalp massage before all the strokes are repeated on the other side of the body.

Keep practising

The neck stroke shown on this page requires practice to perfect. It is a difficult stroke, requiring flexibility of wrist and suppleness of hand to glide over the complex contours of this area and shift pressure from one part of the hand to another in a fluid manner. Once accomplished, it is one of the most satisfying and relaxing strokes of massage.

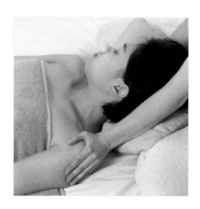

3 Flex your wrist to glide the hand around the joint and lightly behind the shoulder. Then draw your hand up the back of the neck on the side you are massaging.

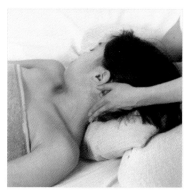

4 Slightly increase the pressure into your fingertips as they glide upwards, so that they gently hook into the neck muscle to stretch it. Mould your hand to the head as it strokes over it and out of the body.

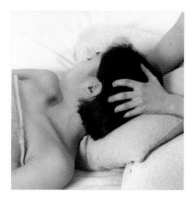

5 Before repeating this sequence of strokes on the other side of the neck, massage this half of the scalp thoroughly to ensure that tension is released fully from the head. Slightly claw your hand and rotate your fingertips in small backward-flowing circles over the scalp.

Soothing strokes for the face

Daily stress can cause the facial muscles to contract, which causes tension. Common habits, such as gritting the teeth or frowning in an effort to resolve problems, increase this tension. Eyestrain can also cause the forehead to tighten and lines to form around the eyes. The strokes of a soothing face massage, described here, can dispel headaches, relax tense muscles and restore physical and mental equilibrium.

The face is one of the most intimate and personal parts of the body, so the quality of touch to this area must always be sensitive and caring. Before beginning, wash your hands. When massaging the face, ensure that your hands are warm and gentle. Mould your hands to its contours and engage both hands equally with each stroke so that its natural symmetry is always defined. Apply the strokes with a calm

Forehead and temples

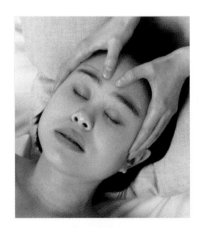

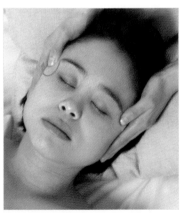

△ A CALMING HOLD *Rest your hands on either side of the jaw, moulding them to its shape. Hold for a few moments until the area begins to warm up.*

△1△ *Place your thumbs at the centre of the forehead, hands gently at the sides. Draw the thumbs steadily out to the sides of the face.*

△2△ *Once they have reached the sides of the face, smoothly circulate your thumb pads over the temples several times.*

and steady pressure, moving consistently from one area of the face to another so that the massage progresses smoothly and avoids any random movements. Try to make the person feel as relaxed as possible by ensuring that they feel comfortable in their surroundings.

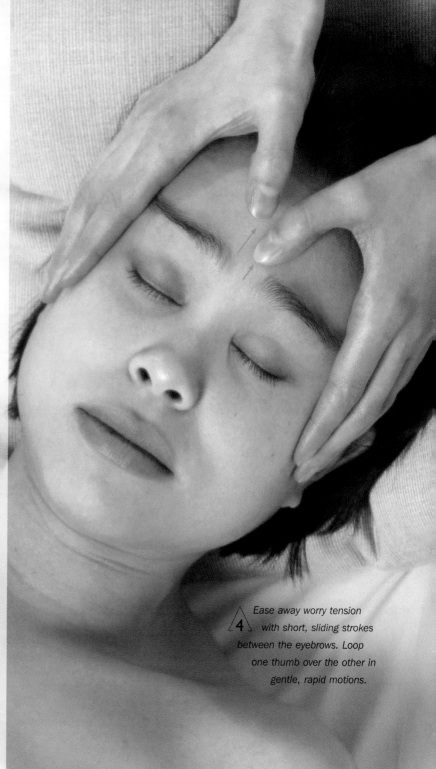

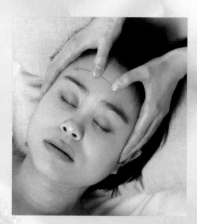

△ **3** Starting slightly higher on the brow, repeat the two previous steps until your thumbs have glided over the entire forehead.

△ **4** Ease away worry tension with short, sliding strokes between the eyebrows. Loop one thumb over the other in gentle, rapid motions.

Eyebrows

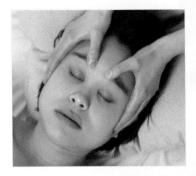

1 Make a smooth, gliding motion over the eyebrows with your thumbs. With your hands resting gently to each side of the face, place your thumb pads on the inner edge of the eyebrows and draw them steadily outwards.

2 As your thumbs slide to the outer edge of the eyebrows, soften the pressure and glide them several times around the temples before drawing your hands up, over and out of the head. Repeat this soothing eyebrow stroke twice more.

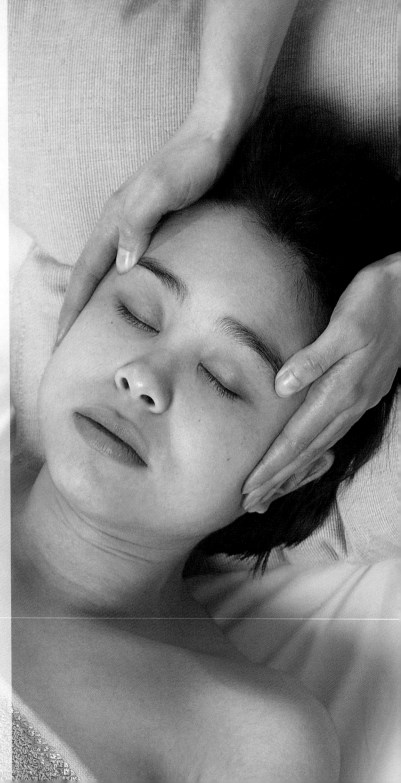

Nose and cheekbones

The steps shown here capture one long sliding motion that uses your thumb pads to stretch down alongside the nose and out under the cheekbones before sweeping your hands over and out of the head.

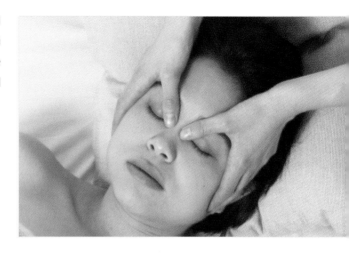

▷ *Start by pressing your thumbs to each side of the bridge of the nose. Glide your thumbs steadily down alongside the nose towards its base before sliding them outwards, directly beneath the cheekbones. The tips of your thumbs should hook lightly into the tissue under the bone.*

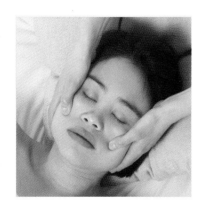

△2 *The area under the cheekbones may be tender so keep the pressure in your thumbs firm but sensitive. As they reach close to the sides of the face, decrease this pressure and relax your hands to mould to the head.*

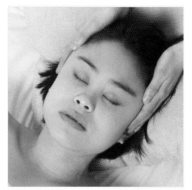

△3 *Without breaking the motion of the stroke, glide both hands smoothly up and over the temples before sweeping them out of the top of the head. Then lightly return your hands to the face to repeat all three stages of the stroke twice more.*

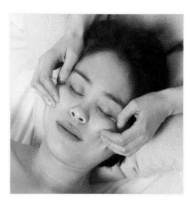

△ RELAXING THE CHEEKS *This stroke will relieve tension from the mouth and jaw. Using your finger-tips make small backward-flowing circles over the fleshy part of the cheeks so that the muscles ripple. Work on one area before moving on to the next.*

Chin and jaw

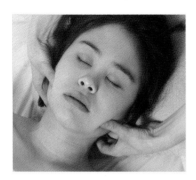

2 With your thumbs looping back over each other, do a rapid succession of downward-sliding thumb strokes on the chin. Support the jaw lightly with your fingers.

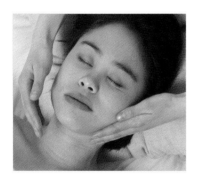

4 EAR MASSAGE Support the ears with your forefingers and move your thumbs over the lobes, before rotating them over the rims. Stroke behind the ears and in the folds. Do not put your fingers into the ear holes.

1 Now use your thumbs to loosen tension from the jaw. Focus on the strong muscles at each edge of the jawbone. Rotate your thumb pads backwards firmly but sensitively into these muscles, encouraging your partner to relax the mouth.

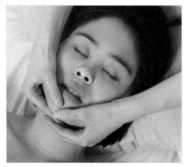

3 Soothe your massage partner by softly caressing one hand after the other at either side of the face. Each hand sweeps up from the chin to glide over the jawbone.

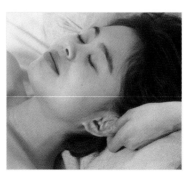

Completing the massage

There are several ways to complete your face massage to accomplish a truly relaxing finish. Comb your fingers gently through the hair several times, as if you are drawing all tension out and away from the body. Then apply a gentle hold, laying your hands softly and symmetrically over the crown of the head for up to one minute, focusing your attention into this contact before withdrawing your hands slowly from the body.

Let your friend rest for five or ten minutes after the massage to fully appreciate and benefit from its effects.

Index

Acknowledgements

The author's thanks go to the whole team at Eddison Sadd for all their hard work on this project, to Sue Atkinson for the beautiful photography and to all the models who took part: Susan Atu, Geoffrey Burton, Alessandra Colangelo, Michael Cooper, Lesley Finn, Mark Gough, Sarah King, Makiko Parsons, Karen Watts and Paul Williams.

EDDISON•SADD EDITIONS

Commissioning Editor	Liz Wheeler
Editors	Nicola Hodgson and Jo Weeks
Proofreader	Michele Turney
Indexer	Dorothy Frame
Art Director	Elaine Partington
Senior Art Editor	Pritty Ramjee
Photographer	Sue Atkinson
Illustrators	Joanna Cameron and Aziz Khan
Production	Karyn Claridge and Charles James